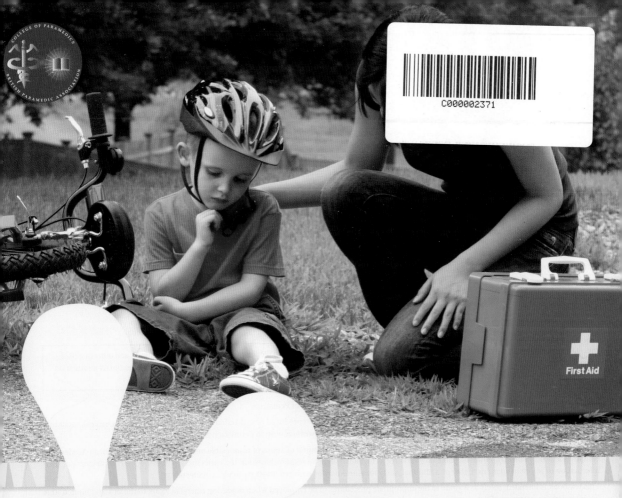

Paediatric First Aid
for Carers and Teachers

American Academy of Pediatrics

DEDICATED TO THE HEALTH OF ALL CHILDREN™

JONES AND BARTLETT PUBLISHERS

Sudbury, Massachusetts

BOSTON   TORONTO   LONDON   SINGAPORE

American Academy of Pediatrics
DEDICATED TO THE HEALTH OF ALL CHILDREN™

Jones and Bartlett Publishers
World Headquarters
40 Tall Pine Drive
Sudbury, MA 01776
info@jbpub.com
www.jbpub.com

Jones and Bartlett Publishers Canada
6339 Ormindale Way
Mississauga, ON L5V 1J2
Canada

Jones and Bartlett Publishers International
Barb House, Barb Mews
London W6 7PA
United Kingdom

American Academy of Pediatrics
141 Northwest Point Boulevard
Post Office Box 927
Elk Grove Village, IL 60009-0927
847-434-4798
www.aap.org

Managing Editor:
Thaddeus Anderson, Manager, Life Support Programs-
    Revised First Edition
Ellen Buerk, MD, MEd, FAAP, AAP Board Reviewer
Robert Perelman, MD, FAAP, Director,
    Department of Education
Wendy Simon, MA, CAE, Director, Life Support Programs
Bonnie Molnar, Life Support Assistant

Jones and Bartlett's books and products are available through
most bookstores and online booksellers. To contact Jones and
Bartlett Publishers directly, call +44(0)1278 723553, fax +44(0)1278
723554, or visit our website, www.jbpub.com.

Substantial discounts on bulk quantities of Jones and Bartlett's publications are available to corporations, professional associations, and other qualified
organizations. For details and specific discount information, contact the special sales department at Jones and Bartlett via the above contact information
or send an email to specialsales@jbpub.com.

The procedures and protocols in this book are based on the most current recommendations of responsible medical sources. The American Academy of
Pediatrics and the publisher, however, make no guarantee as to, and assume no responsibility for, the correctness, sufficiency, or completeness of such
information or recommendations. Other or additional safety measures may be required under particular circumstances.

This textbook is intended, solely as a guide to the appropriate procedures to be employed when rendering emergency care to the sick and injured. It is
not intended as a statement of the procedures required in any particular situation, because circumstances can vary widely from one situation to another.

Additional photographic and illustration credits appear on page 328, which constitutes a continuation of the copyright page.

Production Credits
Chief Executive Officer: Clayton Jones
Chief Operating Officer: Don W. Jones, Jr.
President, Higher Education and Professional Publishing:
    Robert W. Holland, Jr.
V.P., Design and Production: Anne Spencer
V.P., Manufacturing and Inventory Control: Therese Connell
Publisher: Kimberly Brophy
Product Manager: Lorna Downing
Marketing Manager: Brian Rooney
Production Manager: Jenny L. Corriveau

Production Assistant: Tina Chen
Photo Research and Permissions Manager: Kimberly Potvin
Text Design: Anne Spencer
Cover Design: Scott Moden
Cover Image: © Jones and Bartlett Publishers. Photographed by
    Kimberly Potvin.
Composition: Glyph International
Printing and Binding: Imago Group
Cover Printing: Imago Group

Library of Congress Cataloging-in-Publication Data
Paediatric first aid for carers and teachers/American Academy of Pediatrics.— 1st ed.
        p. cm.
    Adapted for use in the U.K.
    ISBN 0-7637-8263-4 (pbk.)
    1. Paediatric emergencies. 2. First aid in illness and injury. 3. CPR (First aid) for children. I. American Academy of Pediatrics.
    RJ370.P4263 2005
    618.92'0025—dc22
                                                            2004026730

6048
Printed in Thailand
13 12 11 10 09   10 9 8 7 6 5 4 3 2 1

Contents

Resource Preview

Paediatric First Aid for Carers and Teachers

Paediatric First Aid for Carers and Teachers (PaedFACTs) can be read either as a stand alone manual or as part of the very successful *PaedFACTs* course, designed to give carers and teachers the education and confidence that they need to effectively care for children.

The *PaedFACTs* course and manual have been carefully written to align with the advice and guidance issues by prominent United Kingdom (UK) bodies. Endorsed by the College of Paramedics in the UK and the American Academy of Pediatrics internationally, any parent, carer, or teacher can be assured of up-to-date and relevant first aid information, approved by professional organisations.

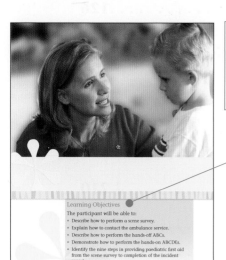

Learning Objectives

Learning objectives are placed at the beginning of each chapter to highlight what students should learn in that chapter.

First Aid Tip

These tips provide instant experience from masters of the trade.

Learning Objectives

The participant will be able to:

- Describe how to perform a scene survey.
- Explain how to contact the ambulance service.
- Describe how to perform the hands-off ABCs.
- Demonstrate how to perform the hands-on ABCDEs.
- Identify the nine steps in providing paediatric first aid from the scene survey to completion of the incident report.

First Aid Tip

As a carer or teacher, you need to remain calm and think before acting. Always handle an ill or injured child gently and avoid any unnecessary movements that might aggravate the problem.

What You Should Know

Before an emergency occurs, all carers and teachers should know how to contact the **ambulance service**. The service provides emergency medical care for an ill or injured child and rapidly transports the child to a medical facility. In the United Kingdom, dialling 999 (or in Europe 112) directly contacts the ambulance service. This number facilitates contact with the ambulance service control room or "Clinical Hub" where trained staff will take your call, dispatch an appropriate resource (ambulance, response car, bike, or helicopter) and may also send a community responder to render immediate aid. The Clinical Hub staff will also provide expert advice prior to the ambulance arriving.

Once you have contacted the ambulance service, provide your location and explain what happened, how many children were involved, and what first aid has been provided. Stay on the line and listen for any additional instructions. Be sure to tell the ambulance service exactly where you and the child are (the specific room within the facility or the location outside). Do not hang up the phone until told to do so by the Emergency Medical Dispatcher (EMD).

Some early education programs have found it helpful to post a list of the items to tell the EMD, including the actual street address and a description of how to get from the street into the facility. In an emergency, it is sometimes difficult to recall familiar information.

It is also important that on field trips and during outside activities, the carer or teacher has access to a telephone, knows how to contact the ambulance service, and knows how to describe the current location of the ill or injured child.

Additional emergency preparations for the facility should include having basic first aid supplies throughout the facility. This should include up-to-date emergency contact information for each child's parent(s) or legal guardian(s). This information should be easily accessible.

Each carer and teacher should know about any child in her care who has a particular health care need. These include allergies to foods or medications, and specific conditions that may complicate first aid care, such as diabetes or asthma. Parent(s) or legal guardian(s) should be asked for permission to make the information about their child's

Did You Know?

This feature provides a better understanding of the topic presented.

First Aid Care

This feature provides short, step-by-step visual reviews of first aid procedures.

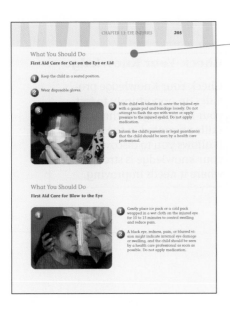

Algorithm

The algorithm is a flowchart designed to reinforce the decision-making process and appropriate first aid care.

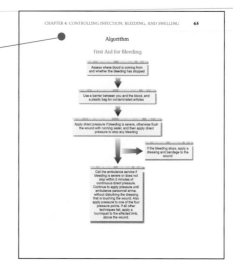

Check Your Knowledge

Check Your Knowledge provides an opportunity to test your knowledge of the first aid skills presented in the chapter. It allows you to discover where your knowledge is strong and where it needs improving.

Acknowledgements

Mark Woolcock, Paramedic
College of Paramedics

We would like to thank the Steering Committee and contributors to *Pediatric First Aid for Teachers and Caregivers.*

Susan Aronson, MD, FAAP, *Chairperson and Editor*
Narbeth, Pennsylvania

Kay Froemming, PNP
Eugene, Oregon

Ronald A. Furnival, MD, FAAP
Salt Lake City, Utah

S. Donald Palmer, MD, FAAP
Magnolia Springs, Alabama

Howard Taras, MD, FAAP
San Diego, California

Alton Thygerson, EdD
Provo, Utah

Rebecca A. Young-Marquardt, MSPH, DrPH
Chapel Hill, North Carolina

Contributors:
Susan Aronson, MD, FAAP
Mark S. Dorfman, MD, FAAP
John M. Flynn, MD, FAAP
Kay Froemming, PNP
Ronald A. Furnival, MD, FAAP
S. Donald Palmer, MD, FAAP
Howard Taras, MD, FAAP
Alton Thygerson, EdD
Michael D. Webb, DDS
Robert A. Wiebe, MD, FAAP
Rebecca A. Young-Marquardt, MSPH, DrPH

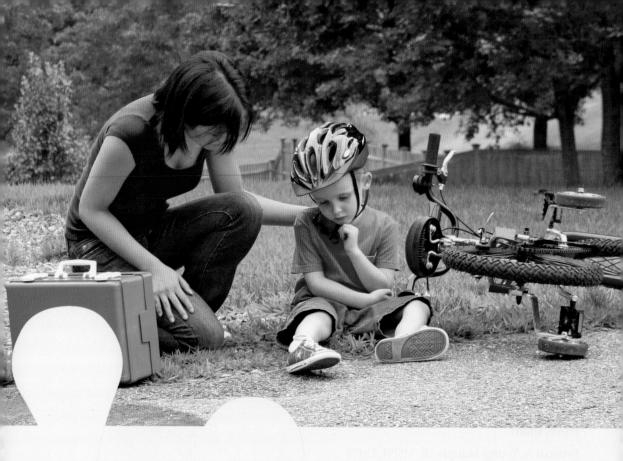

Learning Objectives

The participant will be able to:

- Define paediatric first aid.
- Identify the nine steps involved in providing paediatric first aid.

Chapter 1

What is Paediatric First Aid?

What is Paediatric First Aid?

Carers and teachers need to know what to do when a child is injured or becomes suddenly and severely ill (**Figure 1-1**). Carers can include parents, legal guardians, relatives, and other individuals who care for children. **First aid** is the immediate care given to a suddenly ill or injured child until a medical professional or a parent or legal guardian assumes responsibility for the medical care of the child. First aid is intended to keep the child's medical condition from becoming worse and does not take the place of proper medical treatment. After providing first aid to a child, consultation with the parent(s) or legal guardian(s) and health professionals will determine what, if any, medical treatment is appropriate.

1

Figure 1-1

Carers and teachers need to know what to do when a child is injured or becomes suddenly and severely ill.

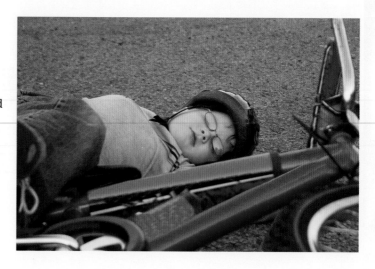

Most injuries that require first aid are not life-threatening. Usually, first aid involves simple, common-sense procedures. However, first aid can sometimes mean the difference between life and death.

All carers and teachers should have paediatric first aid training (**Figure 1-2**). Many people use the term cardio-pulmonary resuscitation (CPR) to refer to all first aid skills. However, this is incorrect. CPR training focuses on what to do when the heart stops beating or when someone cannot breathe. It does not include what to do for all other types of injury or illness situations that might require first aid. For example, it does not teach carers and teachers what to do after a child falls and cuts his knee.

CPR is rarely required for children. For healthy children, the heart typically continues to beat unless the child stops breathing. If breathing stops due to choking, drowning, or a rare heart condition, the heart will eventually stop beating. For this reason, all carers and teachers should at least be trained in management of a blocked airway and rescue breathing. Carers and teachers who care for a child with a rare heart condition or who supervise swimming or wading activities should be trained in CPR, although this training should be offered to anyone who works with children.

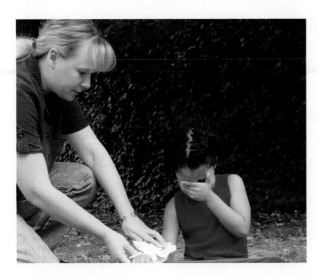

Figure 1-2

All carers and teachers should have paediatric first aid training.

Carers and teachers are expected to provide the same quality of first aid that a layperson with first aid training could provide. Carers and teachers should also be able to obtain prompt help from the ambulance service by dialling 999 or 112. If your facility is in a remote location or participates in activities in remote locations, then more advanced training may be required.

Did You Know?

Situations for which CPR Training for Carers and Teachers is Required:
• Swimming and wading activities
• A child with a rare heart condition

How Will I Learn Paediatric First Aid?

This is the participant manual for the American Academy of Paediatrics (AAP) *Paediatric First Aid for Carers and Teachers (PaedFACTs)* course. It discusses illnesses and injuries that require first aid. The manual is intended as a reference for use during and after the course. It is organized so that topics include the following sections:

Learning Objectives: the expectations of what participants in the *PaedFACTs* course will be able to do after successfully completing their training.

Introduction: an overview of the topic.

What You Should Know: more detailed background information about the topic.

What You Should Look For: the signs and symptoms that carers and teachers need to assess when caring for a child with a particular type of illness or injury.

First Aid Tip

The European Resuscitation Council (ERC) provides guidance on the most up-to-date procedures and techniques for providing basic life support for children who have collapsed.

For the current guidelines, visit the ERC web site at www.erc.edu, or in the United Kingdom visit www.resus.org.uk.

What You Should Do: a reminder about the nine steps in paediatric first aid to follow in every situation that requires first aid, followed by topic-specific instructions for care.

Algorithm: step-by-step first aid instructions.

Check Your Knowledge: multiple-choice questions at the end of the chapter to help you check your understanding of the topic.

You will see that key terms are in **bold type** to help you spot them easily. Also, each topic includes some additional information highlighted in boxes. These may include first aid tips, interesting information, a review of the essential items from the discussion, where to get more information, and illustrations.

As mentioned earlier, each topic will highlight the nine steps in paediatric first aid care. These steps are outlined below and will be discussed in more detail in *Finding Out What is Wrong* (see page 8).

The Nine Steps in Paediatric First Aid:

1 Survey the Scene

Take a brief moment to perform a scene survey to ensure that the scene is safe, to find out who is involved, and to determine what happened.

2 Hands-off ABCs

As you approach the child, perform the hands-off ABCs (Appearance, Breathing, and Circulation) to determine if the ambulance service should be called. It should take 15 to 30 seconds or less.

3 Supervise

Immediately ensure that any other children near the scene are properly supervised.

4 Hands-on ABCDEs

Perform the hands-on ABCDEs (Appearance, Breathing, Circulation, Disability, and Everything else) to determine if the ambulance service should be called and what first aid care is needed.

5 First Aid Care

Provide first aid care appropriate to the injury or illness.

6 Notify

As soon as possible, notify the child's parent(s) or legal guardian(s).

7 Debrief

As soon as possible, talk with the child who received first aid about any concerns he or she may have, and talk with other children who witnessed the injury and first aid procedures.

8 Document

Complete an incident report form.

9 Prevention

Immediately remove or fence off any obvious danger. If this is not possible, report the hazard appropriately and place suitable signage up as an interim measure.

Check Your Knowledge

1. Paediatric first aid is:

   a. Treatment to stop pain and to ensure healing after an injury or in the event of a life-threatening condition.

   b. The immediate care given to an injured or suddenly ill child.

   c. Required only if a child's parent(s) or legal guardian(s) cannot come quickly.

   d. Cardiopulmonary resuscitation.

2. Which of the items listed below is not one of the nine steps involved in paediatric first aid?

   a. Do a quick scene survey to be sure the scene is safe, to know who is involved, and what happened.

   b. Move the child to a comfortable place.

   c. Perform the hands-off ABCs as you approach the child, to see if the ambulance service should be called immediately.

   d. Arrange for supervision of any other children in the group.

3. What kind of people can be defined as carers?

   _____

   _____

   _____

4. What is the purpose of first aid?

   _____

   _____

   _____

Terms

First Aid   The immediate care given to an injured or
                       suddenly ill child until a medical professional
                       or parent(s) or legal guardian(s) assumes re-
                       sponsibility.

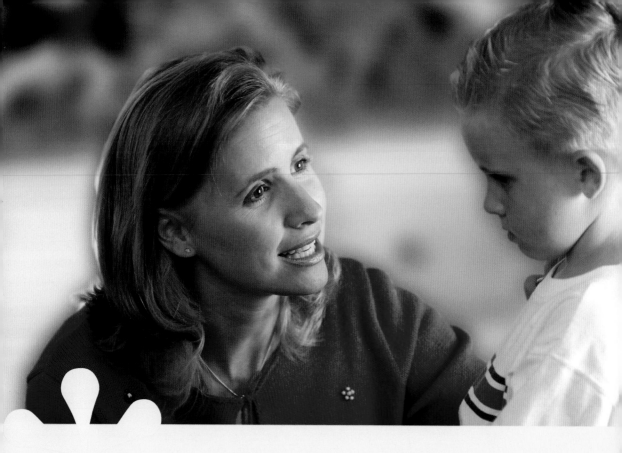

Learning Objectives

The participant will be able to:

- Describe how to perform a scene survey.
- Explain how to contact the ambulance service.
- Describe how to perform the hands-off ABCs.
- Demonstrate how to perform the hands-on ABCDEs.
- Identify the nine steps in providing paediatric first aid from the scene survey to completion of the incident report.

Chapter

2

Finding Out What is Wrong

Finding Out What is Wrong

Introduction

A 3-year-old boy falls from a playground slide and now lies on the ground crying. An 18-month-old girl gets into the cleaning supplies cupboard and is now vomiting. A 3-month-old infant has a fever of 39°C and looks pale. To find out what is wrong with each child, the carer or teacher must practice a calm and methodical approach. This approach will inspire the confidence of the injured child as well as any children witnessing the event.

What You Should Know

Before an emergency occurs, all carers and teachers should know how to contact the **ambulance service**. The service provides emergency medical care for an ill or injured child and rapidly transports the child to a medical facility. In the United Kingdom, dialling 999 (or in Europe 112) directly contacts the ambulance service. This number facilitates contact with the ambulance service control room or "Clinical Hub" where trained staff will take your call, dispatch an appropriate resource (ambulance, response car, bike, or helicopter) and may also send a community responder to render immediate aid. The Clinical Hub staff will also provide expert advice prior to the ambulance arriving.

Once you have contacted the ambulance service, provide your location and explain what happened, how many children were involved, and what first aid has been provided. Stay on the line and listen for any additional instructions. Be sure to tell the ambulance service exactly where you and the child are (the specific room within the facility or the location outside). Do not hang up the phone until told to do so by the Emergency Medical Dispatcher (EMD).

Some early education programs have found it helpful to post a list of the items to tell the EMD, including the actual street address and a description of how to get from the street into the facility. In an emergency, it is sometimes difficult to recall familiar information.

It is also important that on field trips and during outside activities, the carer or teacher has access to a telephone, knows how to contact the ambulance service, and knows how to describe the current location of the ill or injured child.

Additional emergency preparations for the facility should include having basic first aid supplies throughout the facility. This should include up-to-date emergency contact information for each child's parent(s) or legal guardian(s). This information should be easily accessible.

Each carer and teacher should know about any child in her care who has a particular health care need. These include allergies to foods or medications, and specific conditions that may complicate first aid care, such as diabetes or asthma. Parent(s) or legal guardian(s) should be asked for permission to make the information about their child's health needs accessible, so that substitutes and volunteers can be made aware of any needs the child may have.

All facilities which enrol or register children's attendance should keep and maintain an Emergency Information Form (EIF) for every child. While no mandatory template exists, the form must always contain pertinent information about the child's medical history. This must include:

- Medicines, tablets, or ointments used.
- Allergies.
- Sensitivities.
- Homeopathic remedies.
- Initial action required.
- Equipment needs.

A full list of all medical conditions must always be included in the plan. Other information such as emergency contact names and numbers should also feature on this form. The form should ideally be completed by the child's parent or legal guardian and may occasionally contain input from the child's general practitioner (GP) or health care team. In the event of a medical emergency, the EIF should be presented to the ambulance service personnel or be taken to the hospital with the child.

In addition to the EIF, each education program should have a special care plan for any child. The plan should highlight how to care for this child in case of an emergency involving the child or the group, such as the need to evacuate the facility. Developing a special care plan should involve input from the carers and teachers, the child's parent(s) or legal guardian(s), and the child's GP or nurse practitioner.

What You Should Look For

Some conditions warrant calling the ambulance service, while others require prompt medical attention by a health care professional. If in doubt and concerned, you should always call the ambulance service. While some specific conditions should signal a need for immediate medical care, your level of concern is also a good indicator. See Tables 2–1 and 2–2 for a list of conditions that require the ambulance service and situations requiring medical attention.

Table 2–1 When to Call the Ambulance Service

Dial 999 or 112 for the ambulance service immediately for the following:
- Any time you believe a child needs immediate medical treatment.
- Unresponsive child.
- Decreasing responsiveness.
- Excessive drooling, unable to swallow.
- Skin or lips that look purple, blue, or grey.
- Seizures.
- Fever in association with an abnormal ABC (appearance, breathing, or circulation).
- Wounds(s) that will not stop bleeding.
- Burns (see Chapter 11).
- Suddenly spreading purple or red rash.
- Child acting strangely, much less alert or more withdrawn.
- Following a head injury, any of: confusion, headache, vomiting, irritability, unsteadiness, and pain or strange sensation anywhere.
- Increasing severe pain.
- Vomiting blood.
- Large volume of blood in the stools.
- Significant dehydration (sunken features, no tears, not urinating, lethargic).
- Child with severe stiff neck, fever, or headache.
- Hot or cold weather injuries (frostbite, heat exhaustion).
- Multiple children affected by injury or serious illness at same time.

Table 2–2 Situations Requiring Medical Attention

Situations that do not necessarily require an ambulance response, but still need medical attention:
- Fever in any age child who looks more than mildly ill.
- Children younger than 3 months with a temperature of 38°C or higher.
- Children age 3 to 6 months with a temperature of 39°C or higher.
- Severe vomiting and/or diarrhoea.
- A serious cut that may require stitches (i.e., a wound that does not hold together by itself after cleaning).
- Any animal bites that puncture the skin.
- Any bites or stings with spreading local redness and swelling, or evidence of general illness.
- Any medical condition specifically outlined in a child's care plan requiring parental notification.

What You Should Do

The Nine Steps in Paediatric First Aid:

1 **Survey the Scene**

Take a brief moment to perform a scene survey to ensure that the scene is safe, to find out who is involved, and to determine what happened.

2 **Hands-off ABCs**

As you approach the child, perform the hands-off ABCs (Appearance, Breathing, and Circulation) to determine if the ambulance service should be called. It should take 15 to 30 seconds or less.

3 **Supervise**

Immediately ensure that any other children near the scene are properly supervised.

4 **Hands-on ABCDEs**

Perform the hands-on ABCDEs (Appearance, Breathing, Circulation, Disability, and Everything else) to determine if the ambulance service should be called and what first aid care is needed.

5 **First Aid Care**

Provide first aid care appropriate to the injury or illness.

6 **Notify**

As soon as possible, notify the child's parent(s) or legal guardian(s).

7 **Debrief**

As soon as possible, talk with the child who received first aid about any concerns he or she may have, and talk with other children who witnessed the injury and first aid procedures.

8 **Document**

Complete an incident report form.

Prevention

Immediately remove or fence off any obvious danger. If this is not possible, report the hazard appropriately and place suitable signage up as an interim measure.

Finding Out What is Wrong

 Survey the Scene

Begin by taking a quick look at the area surrounding the child. Is the scene safe? Who is involved? What happened? (Safety?-Who?-What?) This quick look should take no more than 15 to 30 seconds.

First, ensure the *safety* of everyone at the scene, including yourself. Look for hazards such as deep water, fire, falling objects, a live electrical wire, or a dangerous animal. Although it is important to quickly reach the child in distress, you must first make sure that the scene is safe. For example, in the case of a fire, you should not rush into a burning building. This is the duty of a properly trained and equipped firefighter. Also, by observing the scene, you may see that more than one child is hurt, although the less seriously injured child may be first to draw your attention by crying. Skipping this step may place more people at risk and delay effective first aid.

Second, find out *who is involved.* Who may also be ill or injured? Are all of the children present? Who needs supervision or comforting? Who can help provide supervision and care for any other children in the group? Are other first aid providers available to help or to contact the ambulance service?

If the scene is not safe and the child must be moved, use the shoulder drag method (**Figure 2-1**). To use this method, place one of your hands on each shoulder, with your forearms along the sides of the head to brace the child's neck during the move. Slowly drag the child to the nearest safe location, while continuing to brace the head and neck. For the child not suspected of having a spinal injury, move the child to a safe place by using the cradle carry for infants or younger children, and the ankle drag for older children (**Figure 2-2A, B**).

For the child who may have fallen, you must always consider the possibility of a spinal injury. If you need to move a child to safety, but a spinal injury is a possibility, do not move the child's head and neck. This may cause spinal cord damage. Encourage injured children not to move if anything hurts. Comforting the ill or injured child without moving her is the safest approach. However, do not forcefully hold a child still. If a child can move all her body parts without pain, there is no need to force the child to hold still.

First Aid Tip

The scene survey involves three tasks:
SAFETY: Is the scene safe?
WHO: Who is involved?
WHAT: What happened?

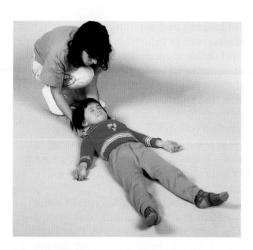

Figure 2-1
Shoulder drag.

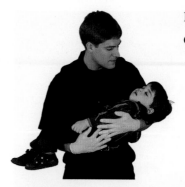

Figure 2-2A
Cradle carry.

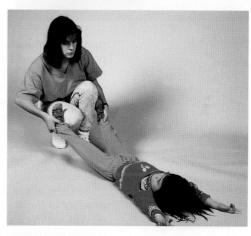

Figure 2-2B
Ankle drag.

Third, find out *what happened.* Identify the possible causes or circumstances of the illness or injury. Did the child fall, and if so, from what height and on what kind of surface? Did the toddler choke on a missing part of a toy? Why is that stray dog near a bleeding child? Did two children run into each other? After completing the three-part scene survey, you will be able to provide safe and effective first aid.

2 Hands-off ABCs

Immediately following the scene survey, perform a check of the child called the **hands-off ABCs: A**ppearance, work of **B**reathing, and **C**irculation (based on skin colour) to see if the ambulance service should be called. The hands-off ABCs are done while you are approaching the ill or injured child, and before you begin care. This is your first chance to look at and listen to the ill or injured child. The hands-off check of the ABCs should take no more than 15 to 30 seconds.

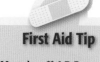

First Aid Tip

Hands-off ABCs
Appearance
Breathing (work of breathing)
Circulation (based on skin colour)

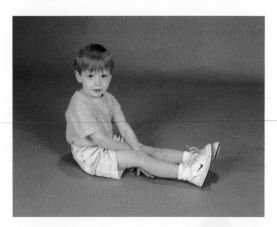

Figure 2-3

Appearance.

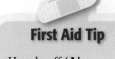

The idea of looking and listening without touching the child who is ill or injured may seem counter to your natural desire to immediately begin to touch and do something for the ill or injured child. However, skipping this step may lead to an incorrect evaluation and management of the child's problem. Use the information from the hands-off ABCs to determine how serious the emergency seems to be and the most appropriate next step in care. How badly is this child injured? What seems to be the child's main problem? Use the hands-off ABCs to decide first, and then act.

With practice, the hands-off ABCs can become automatic. You can practice this look and listen assessment by looking at a healthy child. For instance, when looking at a healthy child, you may notice that she appears active and alert, does not seem to be working harder than usual to breathe, and her skin colour appears normal. Use this as a comparison when looking at a very pale child who is struggling to breathe.

If the hands-off ABCs indicate that the situation requires an ambulance, then ask someone else to call the ambulance service if possible. If this is not possible, and the situation involves a breathing emergency, you should follow the instructions outlined in *Difficulty Breathing.* Provide the EMD with the appropriate information and stay on the line until the EMD says it is okay to hang up.

Be calm while you look at and listen to the child to determine the urgency of the child's problem. Remember, the purpose of the hands-off ABCs is to determine whether to call the ambulance service immediately or to begin providing care.

'A' of the hands-off ABCs is for *Appearance* (**Figure 2-3**). The ill or injured child's appearance is the first and most important observation. The child with an abnormal appearance probably needs urgent care, and you may need to call the ambulance service. **Life-threatening situations** always require calling the ambulance service.

Appearance reflects how well the brain is functioning. How the infant or child interacts with her surroundings is an essential clue. Look at the ill or injured child's alertness, movement, and eye contact. Is the child active with good strength and normal movement, or limp and not moving? Note whether the child seems to respond to someone coming to help when you or another carer or teacher approach her. Does the child make eye contact with you, or does she stare off at nothing in particular?

'B' is for *Breathing.* The child who is working harder to breathe than would be normal for the situation probably needs urgent care, and you need to call the ambulance service. Hands-off evaluation of breathing includes listening for abnormal sounds, looking for an abnormal breathing position, and looking for signs of increased effort.

Is the child making snoring, grunting, wheezing, or gurgling noises with each breath? Is the child's cry or voice weak, hoarse, or muffled? Can the older child only speak a few words at a time? Does the child appear anxious or frightened because of difficulty breathing? Is the child choking?

The child with abnormal breathing often will be more comfortable in an upright position, and may be uncomfortable lying down. A child who is sitting in a **sniffing position,** with her head up and tilted forward, or who is sitting upright and leaning forward with abnormally deep breaths, may be experiencing difficulty breathing. **Nasal flaring,** or flaring of the nostrils is also an indication that the child is having difficulty breathing.

'C' is for *Circulation.* In the hands-off observation, you should note whether the child's skin colour looks unusual. Unusual skin colour for the situation suggests a problem with circulation. It should be considered abnormal, and a sign that you should call the ambulance service to assess the child.

Abnormally light or pale skin colour, or blue colour **(cyanosis)** may indicate a problem with circulation (**Figure 2-4**). When young infants are cold, you may notice a blotchy 'marble' appearance to their skin. This is called **mottling.** A cold infant also may have bluish colour feet and hands. Although pale skin, mottling, and cyanosis (particularly of the hands and feet) may be normal in the infant exposed to cold, it should improve as the infant is warmed up. It is abnormal for a warm child to have these signs. A child whose skin is unusually pink may be overheated or have a rash.

First Aid Tip

Hands-off **'C':**
Circulation
Light or pale skin
Cyanosis (bluish skin colour)
Mottling (blotchy, marble appearance to skin)
Unusually pink skin

3) Supervise

If you are caring for more than one child, you need to arrange for supervision of any other children in the group before you can focus your attention on caring for the ill or injured child. The other children must stay safe. If other carers or teachers are available, ask one of them to take care of the other children, removing them from the area if possible. This will limit the exposure of the other children to the details and involvement in the situation. If you are alone, ask the other children to move away. You might ask them to sit down in a circle. You can tell them you are taking care of the child and you need their help to make the child feel better. You can ask them to sing familiar songs, look at books, or perform any other safe activity that requires minimal involvement from you.

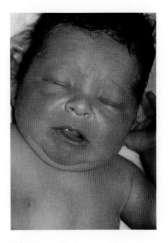

Figure 2-4

Cyanosis.

4) Hands-on ABCDEs

If the hands-off ABCs identify a potentially life-threatening illness or injury, or one that places the child at risk for permanent harm, make sure that you or another adult call the ambulance service immediately. For the child who appears to have an illness or injury that does not require urgent care, you can begin to evaluate and manage the problem with first aid. The hands-on ABCDEs will guide you.

The **hands-on ABCDEs** are a closer look at the ABCs from the hands-off part of the evaluation, adding a 'D' (Disability)

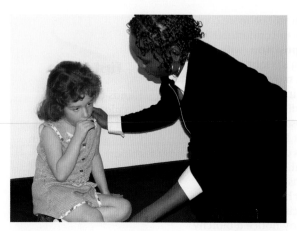

Figure 2-5

Hands-on ABCDEs.

to look at how well the child can move on her own, and 'E' (Everything else) to check the child from head-to-toe for any additional problems. The ABCDEs is a continuation of your initial assessment, once you reach the child, are able to touch the child, and examine the child's response. If at any time during the ABCDEs you discover that the child needs urgent care, you should call the ambulance service immediately.

In the hands-on ABCDEs, 'A' involves a more detailed check of *Appearance.* Does the child respond to gentle touching and stimulation? Is the child's behaviour normal under these circumstances? Does the child awaken and respond in a normal fashion? The infant or child with an abnormal appearance to hands-on ABCDEs may require urgent medical care.

During the hands-on ABCDEs, 'B' is for a more detailed check of *Breathing.* If, in the hands-off ABCs, the child is showing difficulty breathing, the ambulance service should be contacted. If urgent care is not needed, the carer needs to continue to look for further signs of breathing difficulties. Continue to check for abnormal positioning or any changes in breathing patterns, and listen for any abnormal sounds while the child is breathing. If the child is not breathing see Chapter 3, Difficulty Breathing.

'C' of the ABCDEs is for *Circulation,* a hands-on aspect to observations of skin colour. Gently warm the infant or child who has been exposed to cold by adding layers of clothing or a blanket, and then note whether any abnormal colouring of the hands or feet improves. When there is bleeding, continue to monitor circulation while providing first aid. Mottling (blotchy, marble-like appearance to the skin) or cyanosis (blue colour to the skin) requires urgent medical care. Other signs of circulation include breathing, coughing, and movement. If these do not exist, call the ambulance service, and if trained, perform CPR.

'D' stands for *Disability* in the hands-on ABCDEs, which includes observing how well the ill or injured child can move. Does the child sit up, stand up, and move all body parts normally? Does the child squeeze your hand, wiggle her fingers and toes, and move her feet, hands, head, and trunk without stopping because of pain (**Figure 2-5**)? Do not move any body part that the child does not want moved, but gently touch the child to feel if the movements seem normal.

Finally, the hands-on ABCDEs should include 'E' for *Everything else.* Look the child over from head-to-toe. If the ill or injured child can talk, ask if anything hurts, and have the child point to where it hurts. You may need to lift up clothing to look at and gently touch the injured body parts. Does the child with a fever now have a rash? Does the child have reddened or blistered skin from the spilled hot water?

5 First Aid Care

This step is unique to each injury and illness. Your hands-off and hands-on assessments will determine what first aid care you should give to the ill or injured child. The recommended first aid care steps for the various injuries are identified in this text within the various topics.

6 Notify

This step is essential when the person providing first aid is not a parent or legal guardian of the child. Even when medical attention is not required, you should notify the parent(s) or legal guardian(s) about the incident as soon as possible. Sometimes, another person can do this while you care for the child (**Figure 2-6**). Use your emergency contact information to locate the parent(s) or legal guardian(s). While the carer or teacher may not think the child needs care from a health care professional, the parent(s) or legal guardian(s) should have the opportunity to evaluate the situation and decide what to do.

Be calm when notifying the parent(s) or legal guardian(s). Give the facts about what happened to the child. If another child was involved in the event, do not reveal that child's identity. If the ambulance service has been called, let the parent(s) or guardian(s) know where the ambulance service will be taking the child so that they can go to the emergency facility to join the child as soon as possible. Tell the parent(s) or legal guardian(s) about the first aid that the child received, who provided first aid, and who is currently with the child.

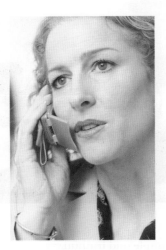

Figure 2-6

Notify the parent(s) or legal guardians as soon as possible.

7 Debrief

After you attend to the needs of the ill or injured child, and the proper individuals have been informed, you need to comfort and address the concerns of the child who received first aid and other children who witnessed the incident and first aid activities. Those who know the children well are best suited to handle this step. The type of comforting and explanation should be developmentally appropriate, and adapted to the temperament and response of the children in the group.

For infants and young toddlers, the approach might involve using a soothing and reassuring tone of voice. You can use a few gently spoken phrases such as "Johnny got hurt. We are making him feel better". Resuming routines as soon as possible helps.

For older children, a carer or teacher can ask the children what they think happened. Listen to what they say, affirm what is correct, and gently correct their misperceptions. Keep explanations simple and truthful (**Figure 2-7**). Minimise sharing graphic details that the children do not bring up themselves. It's a good idea to provide opportunities for children to work through the experience as long as they seem interested in it. Some helpful activities are dramatic play, drawing, storytelling by the children, a non-emergency visit from an ambulance crew, and reading books that relate to the experience. Although an emergency is stressful, the crisis provides an opportunity for children to learn about emergencies and how to cope with them.

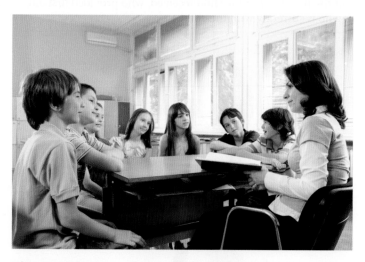

Figure 2-7

Keep explanations simple and truthful.

Since the children who receive or witness first aid in an out-of-home setting may need more comforting at home, be sure to let parent(s) or legal guardian(s) know that there was an emergency during the day. Do not share confidential details, but make the parent(s) or legal guardian(s) aware of what their child may have seen or heard that was unusual for them. Some children may want to talk about the experience at home. Some may show signs or symptoms of having their day's routines upset, such as difficulty sleeping. Others may bring up what they have observed at some other time when the memory of the emergency is triggered by another event. Parent(s) or legal guardian(s) will appreciate being able to understand their children's reactions.

Even seasoned health professionals feel stress when a child has a medical emergency. Talking about what happened and about the feelings related to it can help cope with stress. Plan time to talk.

8 Document

In an education or child care setting, you need to fill out an incident report for any first aid activities. The carer or teacher should carefully document the details of the illness or injury, the first aid provided, the time and details of the call for medical help, the call to the parent(s) or legal guardian(s), and the outcome for the child of the event. Careful documentation is important. Some details are best recorded right away; others may require a day or two before you have the information you need to finish the report. Having a few days to reflect on what happened can be helpful. What you record should always be accurate and objective.

Incident reports help programs for education and child care, parents, legal guardians, insurance companies, and even solicitors document what happened. Administrators who review the forms may help staff think about ways to prevent the situation from happening again. Education programs find it helpful to keep a file of incident reports that they routinely review every 3 to 6 months. A systematic review can identify patterns that suggest a hazardous condition that may not be apparent after a single event.

9 Prevention

Once a child has been safely treated and care for, your attention should turn to whether the same incident could occur again or whether it was a true one-off. If a persistent danger exists, you must take immediate action to either remove the danger or put in place suitable guarding to protect other children. Where a simple or quick solution is not possible, the hazard needs to be reported to someone who has responsibility and ability to remove the hazard. It may be necessary to improvise warning signs until the hazard is eliminated.

Algorithm

Finding Out What is Wrong

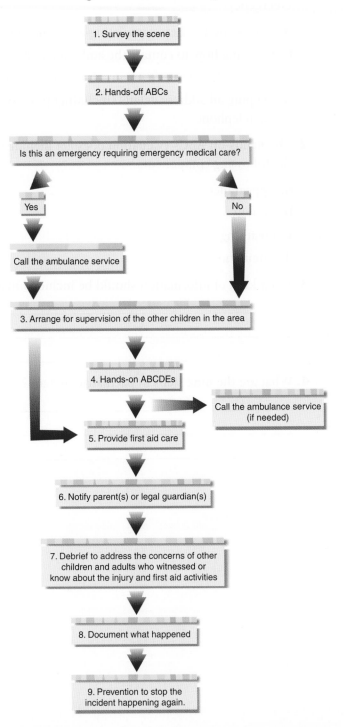

Check Your Knowledge

1. Which of the following is a part of preparing for an emergency?

a. Carers and teachers completing a first aid course

b. Knowing how to contact the ambulance service

c. Keeping the poison centre number by the phones

d. Keeping all address details (including post code) next to the telephone

2. The hands-off ABCs evaluation does *not* include which of the following components?

a. Appearance

b. Activity

c. Breathing

d. Circulation

3. What kind of information should be included in an EIF?

_____

_____

_____

4. What are the nine steps in paediatric first aid?

_____

_____

_____

Terms

Ambulance service	A system that represents the combined efforts of several professionals and agencies to provide emergency medical care.
Cyanosis	Slightly bluish discolouration of the skin.
Hands-off ABCs	The "across the room" assessment performed by someone who is approaching the ill or injured child who is in need of first aid. It includes assessment of appearance, work of breathing, and circulation (based on skin colour).
Hands-on ABCDEs	The assessment done after the hands-off ABCs. It includes a more detailed assessment of appearance, breathing, circulation, disability, and everything else.
Life threatening situations	Any number of conditions caused by illness or injury which require immediate clinical intervention and where a delay may significantly harm the child.
Mottling	A blotchy marble-like appearance to the skin.
Nasal flaring	When infants and young children are working hard to breathe, they often will open or flare their nasal passages with each attempt to breathe air in.
Sniffing position	When the child sits with head slightly elevated and is leaning forward as if she were sniffing a flower.

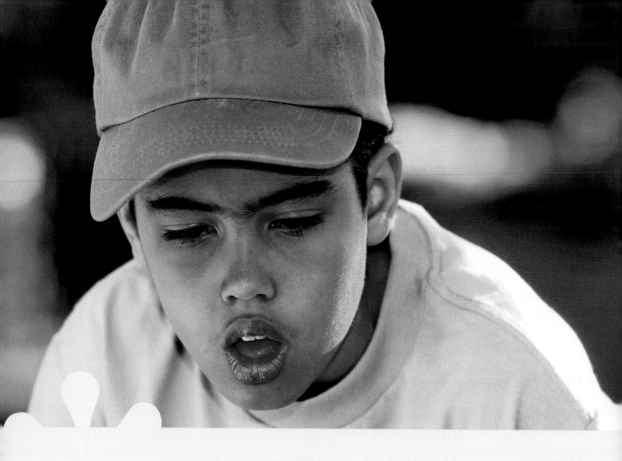

Learning Objectives

The participant will be able to:

- Recognise an infant or child who is unresponsive and call the ambulance service.
- Recognise an infant who is having difficulty breathing and determine if management of a blocked airway is needed.
- Recognise a child who is having difficulty breathing and determine if rescue breathing is needed.
- Demonstrate the management of a blocked airway on an infant manikin.
- Demonstrate the management of a blocked airway on a child manikin.
- Demonstrate rescue breathing.

Chapter

3

Difficulty Breathing

Difficulty Breathing

Introduction

The body needs oxygen to live. Oxygen enters the body through the lungs, where it passes into the blood. The heart circulates the oxygen-rich blood into every cell in the body, and the most demanding user of oxygen is the brain. The brain can survive for only a few minutes without oxygen before brain damage is likely to occur (**Figure 3-1**). This is why **respiratory arrest** (when breathing stops) and **cardiac arrest** (when the heart stops) are the most urgent life-threatening emergencies.

Figure 3-1

Brain damage occurs quickly if oxygen is not delivered.

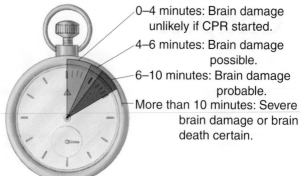

0–4 minutes: Brain damage unlikely if CPR started.

4–6 minutes: Brain damage possible.

6–10 minutes: Brain damage probable.

More than 10 minutes: Severe brain damage or brain death certain.

What You Should Know

Cardiac arrest rarely occurs in children. For most children, the heart is a healthy, strong muscle that pumps blood through the body. When a child's heart stops beating, it is seldom caused by a problem within the heart. Rather, it is usually the result of an injury that first caused the child to be unable to breathe. The most common causes for breathing problems in infants and young children are respiratory infection, choking, and drowning. Asthma and allergic reactions may also cause swelling in the airway that can lead to difficulty breathing (**Figure 3-2**).

Figure 3-2

The respiratory system.

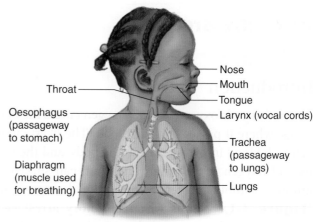

Throat

Oesophagus (passageway to stomach)

Diaphragm (muscle used for breathing)

Nose

Mouth

Tongue

Larynx (vocal cords)

Trachea (passageway to lungs)

Lungs

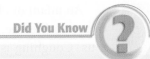

Did You Know

Except for children with cardiac problems, or in cases of drowning, a child's heart typically does not stop beating unless the child first stops breathing. Therefore, cardiopulmonary resuscitation (CPR) training is strongly recommended for facilities that enroll children with conditions that may result in cardiac arrest or those programs that have higher risk activities such as swimming. All carers in early education and child care settings should learn how to manage a blocked airway and provide rescue breathing.

Quickly removing an object that is blocking the airway so that air can get into the lungs is called management of a blocked airway. Breathing cannot occur if the airway is blocked. Getting air back into the lungs of a child who is not breathing is called **rescue breathing**. Management of a blocked airway and rescue breathing are the most important and critical skills that anyone who cares for children of any age can learn. A child may die unless management of a blocked airway and rescue breathing are started while waiting for ambulance personnel to arrive.

What You Should Look For

Choking is a preventable, but common problem. A child may put a coin, button, or small toy in his mouth, or bite a balloon and take a breath, sucking the object into his airway. An object lodged in the airway can cause a partial or complete blockage. A completely blocked airway prevents oxygen from entering the lungs. An infant or child with a completely blocked airway will become unresponsive within minutes if the object is not removed. When a child has a completely blocked airway, he is generally unable to cry, speak, breathe, or cough. When you ask an older child who has a blocked airway, "Can you speak?" he is unable to respond verbally. An older child who is choking may instinctively reach and clutch his neck, to signal that he is choking. This motion is known as the **universal distress signal** for choking (**Figure 3-3**).

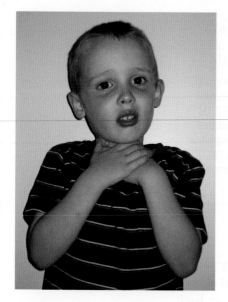

Figure 3-3

Universal dis-
tress signal.

An infant or child with a partially blocked airway continues to breathe, but will usually be coughing and anxious. Coughing is the body's way of removing what feels
like a foreign object. This feeling occurs when there is
swelling, irritation, or mucus anywhere in the airway. This
is why people often cough when they have sinusitis or a
runny nose. When there is an object in the airway, forceful
coughing is more effective than anything anyone else can
do to get the object to move up and out of the airway.

A child with difficulty breathing may also have respiratory distress. Respiratory distress most commonly occurs in
children with asthma or wheezing. Wheezing can come on
suddenly. A child who is known to have wheezing problems
may have a prescription medicine that can help relieve
wheezing, such as blue or brown inhalers. Carers and
teachers should follow the instructions for using this medicine without delay.

Children with asthma or an airway infection who are working
hard to breathe may tire and stop breathing. This requires an immediate response from the ambulance service. It is always best to call
the ambulance crew before a child gets to this stage; early access to
999 or 112 is absolutely essential.

When a child has been submerged in water and is not breathing, this is called drowning. The non-breathing child who has suffered a suffocation injury from submersion in water will need rescue breathing while the ambulance is en route.

The most important signs to recognise are those that show you
that a child is working hard to breathe. You may see some of the
signs of difficulty breathing:

- Drooling (unrelated to teething) occurs when a child is
  unable to swallow saliva either because of swelling in the
  back of his throat or because it is hard to swallow saliva
  while leaning forward and working hard to breathe.
- Head bobbing may occur when the child is working hard to
  breathe. The strong contraction of the neck muscles may
  move the head and pull up on the chest.

- **Nasal flaring** occurs when a child automatically opens or flares his nasal passages with each attempt to breathe air in, trying to get as much air in as possible (**Figure 3-4**).
- **Sniffing position** is the way a child lifts his head slightly and leans forward as if he is sniffing a flower while trying to get more air into his lungs.
- **Tripod position** is the way a child will lean forward with outstretched arms, usually placed on top of the knees to make the best use of respiratory muscles.
- **Wheezing** is the production of whistling sounds when the child breathes. This sound is a result of swelling or blockage of the small tubes (bronchioles) in the lungs.

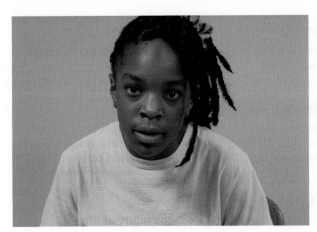

Figure 3-4

Nasal flaring.

What You Should Do

The Nine Steps in Paediatric First Aid:

1 Survey the Scene

Take a brief moment to perform a scene survey to ensure that the scene is safe, to find out who is involved, and to determine what happened.

2 Hands-off ABCs

As you approach the child, perform the hands-off ABCs (Appearance, Breathing, and Circulation) to determine if the ambulance service should be called. It should take 15 to 30 seconds or less.

3 Supervise

Immediately ensure that any other children near the scene are properly supervised.

4 Hands-on ABCDEs

Perform the hands-on ABCDEs (Appearance, Breathing, Circulation, Disability, and Everything else) to determine if the ambulance service should be called and what first aid care is needed.

5 First Aid Care

Provide first aid care appropriate to the injury or illness.

6 Notify

As soon as possible, notify the child's parent(s) or legal guardian(s).

7 Debrief

As soon as possible, talk with the child who received first aid about any concerns he or she may have, and talk with other children who witnessed the injury and first aid procedures.

8 Document

Complete an incident report form.

9 **Prevention**

Immediately remove or fence off any obvious danger. If this is not possible, report the hazard appropriately and place suitable signage up as an interim measure.

For any emergency situation, follow the nine steps for paediatric first aid. When you see that the child is having difficulty breathing, you must call the ambulance service and provide immediate care for the breathing problem before you do anything else.

What You Should Do

First Aid for a Responsive Infant or Child with a Blocked Airway

Do not start management of a partially blocked airway if the infant or child can breathe, cry, speak, or cough. A good cough is more effective than anything you can do to clear the airway. If a child cannot breathe, cough, or make a normal voice sound and is still responsive, have someone call the ambulance service as you begin first aid care. If you are alone, call the ambulance service after providing 1 minute of first aid care.

First Aid Tip

Encouraging the child to give a good cough is one of the most effective ways of clearing a blockage in their airway.

The technique for managing a blocked airway in a responsive infant (less than 1 year of age) consists of repeating a combination of five back blows and five chests thrusts. To perform back blows on an infant, turn the infant's head down on your forearm, with his feet up toward your shoulder. Place your hand around the infant's jaw and neck. The infant's head should be at a height lower than your trunk. Rest your arm against your thigh for support. Using the heel of your hand, give five quick, sharp back blows between the infant's shoulder blades (**Figure 3-5**).

Figure 3-5

Using the heel of your
hand, give five quick,
sharp back blows
between the infant's
shoulder blades.

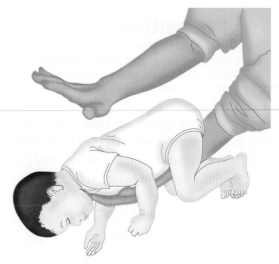

Did You Know ?

Back blows are used for responsive choking infants because the infant's chest is small and flexible. Giving back blows with the infant's head down may cause enough chest movement that, in combination with gravity, may move the foreign object toward the
mouth. If the object is moved a little, the infant may be able to
cough the object out.

After doing five back blows, give five chest thrusts. To perform
chest thrusts on an infant, place your free hand on the back of the
infant's head and neck, keeping the other hand that is supporting the
head in place. Use both hands and forearms (one on the back and
one on the front of the infant's body) to firmly hold the infant's body
as you turn the infant over (**Figure 3-6**). Once turned onto his
back, the infant should be resting on your arm, with your arm
against your thigh. The infant's head should be lower than your
trunk. Place two fingers on the infant's breastbone slightly below the
nipple line. Avoid the bottom tip of the breastbone. Give five chest
thrusts; these are similar to CPR chest compressions but are sharper
in nature and delivered slightly slower.

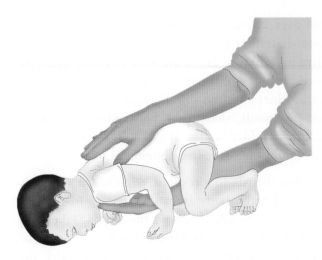

Figure 3-6

Use both hands and forearms (one on the back and one on the front of the infant's body) to firmly hold the infant's body as you turn the infant over.

Check inside the infant's mouth after you do the chest thrusts. If you see the foreign object, carefully remove it. Do not attempt a blind finger sweep to remove an object that you cannot see, since you might push it deeper. Continue alternating back blows and chest thrusts, and looking for an object until the ambulance arrives, the object is removed, or the infant becomes unresponsive.

First Aid Tip

For a responsive infant who is choking:
1. Call the ambulance service*
2. Give five back blows
3. Give five chest thrusts
4. Check the mouth
5. Continue alternating five back blows with five chest thrusts until the ambulance service arrives, the foreign body is removed, or the infant becomes unresponsive

*If you are alone, provide 1 minute of first aid and then call the ambulance service.

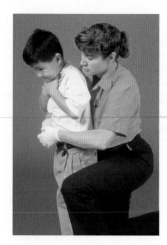

Figure 3-7

Continue abdominal thrusts until the ambulance arrives, the object is removed, or the child becomes unresponsive.

For any child over 1 year of age who is choking, you should call for help immediately. If coughing has not relieved the obstruction, give five back blows. These are most effective when the child is positioned head down; small children can be placed over your knees whereas older children should be placed in a forward-leaning position. Five swift, sharp back blows should be delivered in between the shoulder blades. If this fails to dislodge the obstruction, you should then give five abdominal thrusts.

Giving abdominal thrusts to a responsive child who is choking can dislodge the foreign body from the airway. To give abdominal thrusts, position yourself behind the child. Make a fist and place it just above the navel, and below the breastbone. Pull the child close to you and with your closed fist, give quick upward and inward thrusts to the child's abdomen. Continue abdominal thrusts until the ambulance service arrives, the object is removed, or the child becomes unresponsive (**Figure 3-7**).

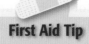

First Aid Tip

For a responsive child over 1 year of age who is choking:
- Call for help*
- Give five back blows
- Give five abdominal thrusts
- Continue until the ambulance arrives, the object is removed, or the child becomes unresponsive.

*If you are alone, provide 1 minute of first aid and then call the ambulance service.

What You Should Do

First Aid for an Infant or Child Who is Unresponsive and Not Breathing

Rescue breathing is the technique to use when the infant or child is not breathing. If an infant or child is unresponsive and is not breathing or is choking and becomes unresponsive, you need to begin rescue breathing. The steps for rescue breathing include:

1. **Check for responsiveness:** The first step is to determine if you need to do rescue breathing. You do not use rescue breathing on a responsive infant or child. Gently tap the infant's or child's body and shout, "Are you okay?" (**Figure 3-8**).

2. **Call for help:** If an infant or child is unresponsive, shout for help and ask someone to call 999 or 112. If you are alone, perform 1 minute of care before going for help. It may be possible to carry an infant or small child with you whilst summoning help (**Figure 3-9**).

3. **Open the airway:** Use the head-tilt/chin-lift method (**Figure 3-10A**). To do this, place your hand on the infant's or child's forehead and tilt the head back slightly. Place the fingers of your other hand under the chin and lift gently; avoid pressing on the soft tissues under the jaw. If you suspect a possible spinal injury, use the jaw-thrust technique without head-tilt to open the airway (**Figure 3-10B**). To do this, stabilise the head and place your fingers behind the angles of the lower jaw on each side of the head. Move the lower jaw forward without moving or tilting the head backward.

4. **LOOK, LISTEN and FEEL for breathing:** See if the chest and abdomen are rising and falling as they normally do when an infant or child is breathing (**Figure 3-11**). Place your ear over the infant's or child's mouth and nose while keeping the airway open and listen and feel for breathing. With your ear over the face, continue to look at the chest and abdomen to check for rise and fall with breathing for no more than 10 seconds.

5. **Look in the mouth for an object:** Look for an object that you can remove easily. Do not perform a blind finger sweep of the mouth. Your attempts could push the object into the airway.

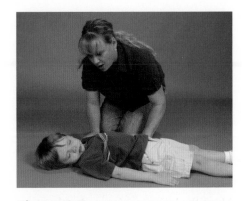

Figure 3-8

Check for responsiveness.

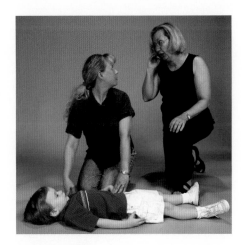

Figure 3-9

Call the ambulance service.

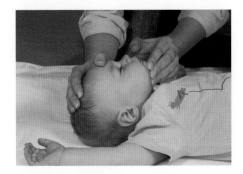

Figure 3-10A

The head-tilt/chin-lift method.

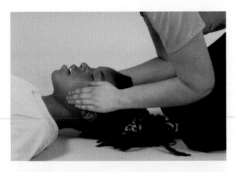

Figure 3-10B

Move the lower jaw forward without moving or tilting the head backward.

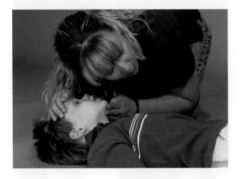

Figure 3-11

LOOK, LISTEN and FEEL for breathing.

6. **Give rescue breaths.** If you do not see an object in the infant's or child's mouth and he does not start to breathe after opening the airway, give five initial rescue breaths (1 second per breath), enough so that you can see the chest rise and fall. The difference between the way you give rescue breaths for a child and for an infant is the way in which you seal your mouth over the airway to breathe air into the lungs. For the infant, you tilt the head back and seal your mouth over the infant's nose and mouth, and breathe into the nose and mouth (**Figure 3-12A**). For the child, you may have difficulty sealing your mouth around the child's mouth and nose (**Figure 3-12B**). Instead, pinch the child's nose, and then breathe into the child's mouth. Allow air to flow out of the chest after each breath. Each breath should take 1 second for air entry and about the same amount of time to allow for the air to flow out of the chest. If the chest does not rise and fall with the attempt to give the first breath, reposition the head and chin to open the airway and attempt to give another breath. If all five breaths are unsuccessful, begin treatment for an airway obstuction (previously discussed).

7. **Begin alternating 30 chest compressions and two rescue breaths.** Compress the chest of an infant or child approximately $1/3$ of the depth of the chest

Figure 3-12A

For the infant, you tilt the head back and seal your mouth over the infant's nose and mouth, and breathe into the nose and mouth.

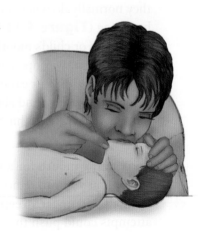

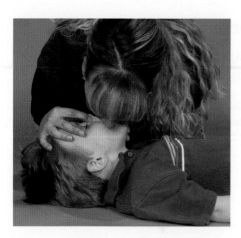

Figure 3-12B

For the child, you may have difficulty sealing your mouth around the child's mouth and nose. Pinch the child's nose and then breathe into the child's mouth.

(**Figure 3-13A, B**). Continue providing rescue breaths and chest compressions until the infant or child begins breathing or the ambulance service arrives.

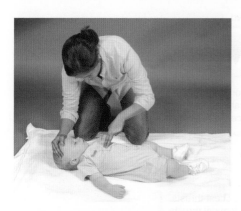

Figure 3-13A

Compress the chest of an infant approximately $1/3$ of the depth of the chest.

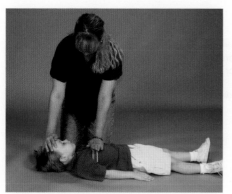

Figure 3-13B

Compress the chest of a child approximately $1/3$ of the depth of the chest.

Algorithm

First Aid for a Responsive Infant or Child with a Blocked Airway

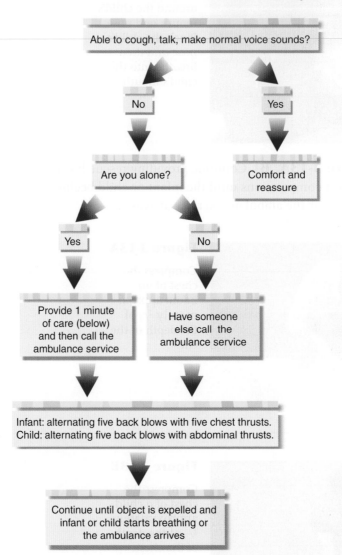

Able to cough, talk, make normal voice sounds?

No

Yes

Are you alone?

Comfort and reassure

Yes

No

Provide 1 minute of care (below) and then call the ambulance service

Have someone else call the ambulance service

Infant: alternating five back blows with five chest thrusts.
Child: alternating five back blows with abdominal thrusts.

Continue until object is expelled and infant or child starts breathing or the ambulance arrives

First Aid for an Infant or Child Who is Unresponsive and Not Breathing

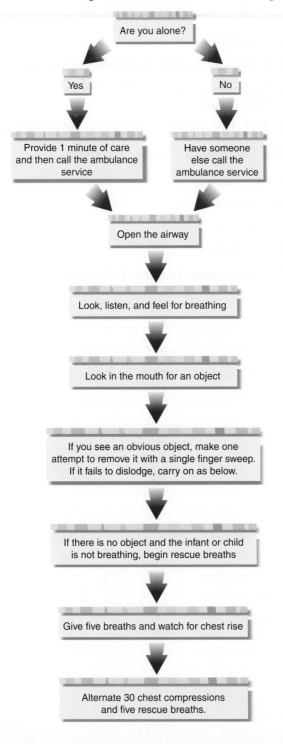

Are you alone?

Yes

No

Provide 1 minute of care and then call the ambulance service

Have someone else call the ambulance service

Open the airway

Look, listen, and feel for breathing

Look in the mouth for an object

If you see an obvious object, make one attempt to remove it with a single finger sweep. If it fails to dislodge, carry on as below.

If there is no object and the infant or child is not breathing, begin rescue breaths

Give five breaths and watch for chest rise

Alternate 30 chest compressions and five rescue breaths.

Check Your Knowledge

1. When you are alone and caring for an unresponsive choking child with a blocked airway, call the ambulance service:

   a. Immediately.

   b. As soon as the object of obstruction is removed.

   c. After approximately 1 minute of performing first aid care.

   d. If 30 chest compressions do not remove the obstruction.

2. How long should a rescue breath take?

   a. 1 second.

   b. 2 seconds.

   c. 3 seconds.

   d. 4 seconds.

3. What are common causes of a blocked airway in children?

   _____

   _____

   _____

4. What should your actions be for a child who is choking?

   _____

   _____

   _____

Terms

Cardiac arrest	When the heart stops beating.
Nasal flaring	Enlarging of the opening of the nostrils.
Rescue breathing	The act of breathing for a person who is not breathing.
Respiratory arrest	When breathing stops.
Sniffing position	A position children may assume when working hard to breathe; their heads are slightly elevated and they lean forward as if they are sniffing a flower.
Tripod position	The way a child will sit up, placing his arms in front of his chest and out to his side to make the best use of his respiratory muscles.
Universal distress signal	The hands around the throat is the universal distress signal for choking.
Wheezing	A whistling sound made by a child with swelling or blockage of chest tubes.

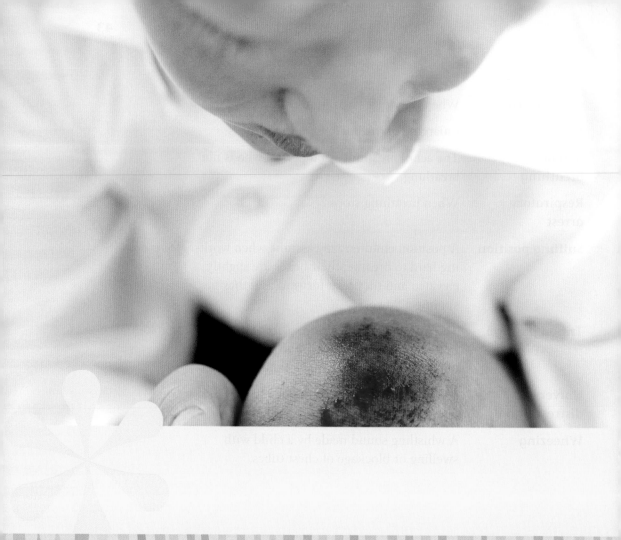

Learning Objectives

The participant will be able to:

- Describe Standard Precautions and Universal Precautions.
- Recognise abrasions, contusions, incisions, lacerations, and puncture wounds.
- Demonstrate how to apply direct pressure to a bleeding wound.
- Describe the appropriate first aid for abrasions, contusions, incisions, lacerations, blisters, bruises, and puncture wounds.
- Demonstrate how to control a nosebleed.

Chapter

4

Controlling Infection, Bleeding, and Swelling

Controlling Infection

Introduction

Infections are caused by viruses, bacteria, and other germs. Infections can be passed from one person to another. Knowing how germs are transmitted and how to protect against infection while performing first aid will enable you to act wisely and with confidence. While caring for wounds, you need to know how to prevent infection of the wound and how to handle body fluids to protect yourself from infection.

What You Should Know

Controlling the spread of infection requires protecting yourself against exposure to germs and reducing the number of germs in the environment. When the skin has been opened by an injury, germs can enter this opening and start to grow. Reducing the number of germs in a wound helps prevent infection. You can reduce the number of germs by rinsing wounds with soap and running water as soon as possible. You must be sure to control bleeding first, and then rinse out a wound to remove dirt and germs. Generally, except for nosebleeds and wounds that are bleeding freely, prompt rinsing of an open wound with soap and running water is appropriate first aid to reduce the number of germs that can cause infection. The sooner the germs are rinsed out of a wound, the better. Germs multiply very rapidly in a wound and can soon overwhelm the body's defences against infection.

When body fluids contact an object that others might touch, the body fluids must be removed by cleaning with detergent and rinsing with water. This helps to remove the source of infection, although some germs will remain. To further reduce the number of germs left behind on the visibly clean surface, use a disinfectant. This two-step process makes infection from body fluids unlikely.

Standard Precautions and **Universal Precautions** describe actions developed by the Centres for Disease Control and Prevention (CDC) and the Occupational Safety and Health Administration (OSHA) to help protect people from infections transferred through body fluids. Standard Precautions are the measures required to protect against contact with any type of body fluid, except sweat. Universal Precautions are the protective measures that apply only to blood, and body fluids that might contain blood.

Hand washing after cleaning and sanitising is essential (**Figure 4-1**). Wearing gloves or using other barriers are not a substitute for washing your hands with soap and running water after a possible exposure to a body fluid. Individuals should wash their hands carefully after possible contact with germs, whether or not barriers were used. Using a barrier reduces, but does not totally eliminate, contact with body fluids.

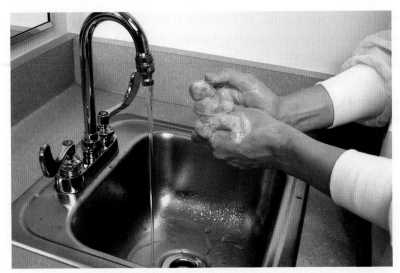

Figure 4-1

Hand washing
is essential.

As mentioned, universal precautions are guidelines designed to protect persons from exposure to potentially infectious diseases spread by blood and body fluids. It is important to protect yourself when handling any body fluid and to treat all fluids as potentially harmful. Remember that universal precautions are designed to protect both the carer and the child.

Typically, the minimally accepted universal precautions include wearing protective gloves when treating any ill or injured child. Gloves are meant to provide a barrier between your skin and any potentially harmful body fluid(s).

Additional precautions also include eye protection (goggles) for splashing fluids or face shields (masks) when coughing and sneezing are present.

The need for such precautions has come about with the increased awareness of HIV/AIDS. Human immunodeficiency virus (HIV) is a virus that causes acquired immune deficiency syndrome (AIDS). Children with HIV are considered to be HIV positive and are never "cured" but do not always develop AIDS. Children who are HIV positive can lead normal lives and may never develop AIDS or complications.

HIV is transmitted through body fluids and primarily through sexual intercourse, breastfeeding, childbirth, sharing of needles, and blood transfusions. HIV is not transmitted by: saliva, tears, sweat, faeces or urine; hugging; kissing; shaking hands; insect bites; or sharing toilets with an HIV positive child.

Remember to protect yourself prior to caring for any ill or injured child. Use the universal precautions and you will significantly decrease the risk of exposure to diseases.

First Aid Tip

Reducing contact with germs can help to control the spread of germs and prevent infection. Using the following barriers can help to reduce the exposure of staff and children to germs:
- Non-porous gloves (such as non-latex medical exam gloves or vinyl gloves) (**Figure 4-2**)
- Disposable changing mats/cover for nappy changes
- Disposable towels for cleaning-up and disinfecting surfaces
- Non-porous surfaces that can be cleaned and disinfected
- Clothing to prevent contact of your skin with the body fluids of someone else, especially when blood might be involved and you do not have gloves
- Plastic bags to store contaminated articles until they can be thrown away

Figure 4-2

Gloves are a barrier against germs.

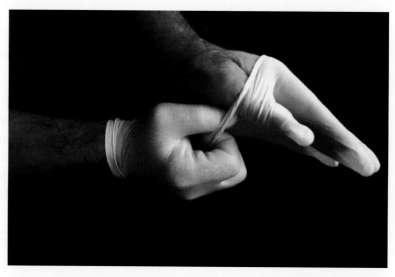

What You Should Look For

When a child has been injured, you need to look for places where the skin has been cut or where tissues have been injured. Tissue injury comes from some force pressing hard on a body part, twisting or pinching the skin or other tissues. Bleeding, bruising, swelling, or pain may indicate tissue injury. If the injury has opened the skin, you may come in contact with blood.

Having cuts or open sores on your own hands increases your risk of getting an infection from contact with germs from surfaces and from a child's body fluids. If you have cuts or sores on your hands, you need to protect these openings with clean coverings (e.g., a bandage) and wear non-porous gloves when handling body fluids.

What You Should Do

Procedure for Standard Precautions When Cleaning Up Body Fluids

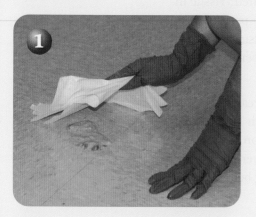

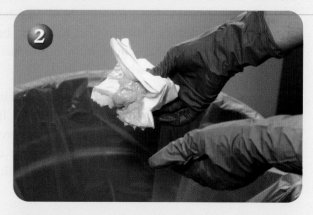

1 Use non-porous gloves and whatever tools (e.g., paper towels, tissues, rags, mop) you have to wipe up the spill. Try to use disposable tools to minimise the need to do further cleaning and disinfecting. Avoid spreading the spilled body fluid.

2 Put all tools (e.g., paper towels, tissues, rags, mops) that you used to wipe up the spill into a recognised clinical waste style bag. If these are not available, place all into a plastic bag. Secure the plastic bag and place it into another bag which is secured and ready for disposal.

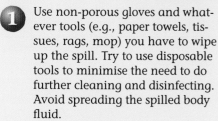

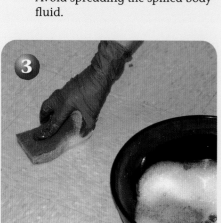

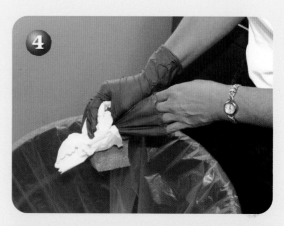

3 Use a solution of water and chlorine tablets dissolved to 10,000 ppm to clean all surfaces in contact with the spill.

4 Put contaminated cleaning material in a plastic bag with a secure tie for disposal. This can be the same plastic bag you used for the tools from wiping up the spill. Allow all surfaces to air dry.

Bleeding

What You Should Know

When the skin is cut and a blood vessel of any size is broken, bleeding occurs. The seriousness of the injury is determined by the depth of the cut, the type of blood vessels damaged, and the amount of bleeding that occurs. The most severe bleeding is from **arteries**, which are large, deep, and well-protected blood vessels. Injury to an artery is serious. Large amounts of blood can be lost from arteries in a short amount of time. If arterial bleeding is not controlled, the child will go into shock. Shock is a condition when the blood cannot deliver oxygen to the body's cells. A child who becomes shocked through loss of blood will look very pale, have a fast breathing rate, and a fast pulse. This is a potentially life-threatening situation. Applying pressure to a wound with your hand or with a firmly applied dressing is called **direct pressure** (**Figure 4-3**). In extreme cases where you are unable to stem the flow of blood, it is recommended to use a **tourniquet** on the affected limb.

Veins are blood vessels that are located closer to the surface of the skin. Although a vein can bleed heavily, the bleeding can usually be controlled with simple first aid measures. Direct pressure works well for controlling bleeding from veins.

First Aid Tip

The seriousness of the injury is determined by the depth of the cut, the type of blood vessels damaged, and the amount of blood loss.

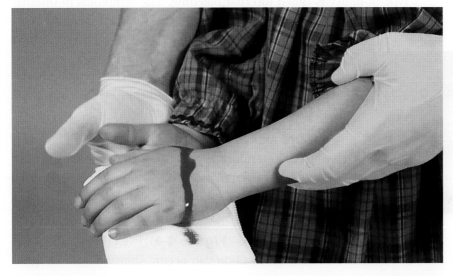

Figure 4-3

Applying direct pressure.

Tiny blood vessels located throughout the body are called **capillaries**. There are hundreds of thousands of capillaries throughout the body. When capillaries are broken, bleeding is easy to control. Direct pressure stops bleeding from capillaries quickly.

Some parts of the body have more blood vessels than others. For example, the head and face have more blood vessels in a given area than the finger. That is why a cut on the head or face bleeds more than a cut on a finger.

Injuries that occur deep in the chest, abdomen, or in the brain may be associated with bleeding in tissues far below the skin. This type of injury is called **internal bleeding**. The symptoms of internal bleeding vary with the type of injury and the body part involved. Usually, the person with internal bleeding feels severe pain and looks very ill. If you suspect that a child may have internal bleeding, call the ambulance service immediately. Attempt to keep the child calm while waiting for the ambulance service to arrive.

If the skin is broken, the wound is called an **open wound**. Common types of open wounds include scrapes (abrasions), cuts (lacerations, incisions), broken blisters, punctures, and nosebleeds.

Abrasions occur when the top layer of skin is removed, with little blood loss (**Figure 4-4**). Even though abrasions are not life-threatening, infection can occur. Abrasions can be quite

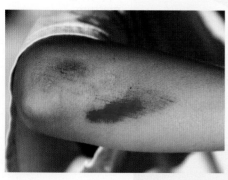

Figure 4-4

Abrasion.

painful. Many nerve endings may be exposed with the loss of the top layer of skin. An example of an abrasion is a scraped elbow.

A **laceration** is a break in the skin caused by blunt force. The skin has been burst rather than cut. It will look more ragged than an incised wound. An **incision** or cut is a break in the skin caused by something with a sharp edge such as a knife, razor blade, or glass (**Figure 4-5**). These wounds look neat and tend to be relatively easy to close.

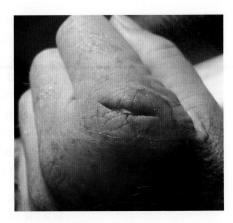

Figure 4-5

Incision.

A **blister** is a collection of fluid in a bubble underneath the skin. These can be small or large. Generally, if the skin over a blister is not broken, the fluid inside the blister is sterile.

A **puncture** is a small hole made in the skin, which may be either deep or shallow (**Figure 4-6**). Puncture wounds usually bleed very little. Puncture wounds have a high risk of infection because it is hard to wash out the germs in the hole that the penetrating object made in the skin. An example of a puncture wound is a splinter.

An avulsion is a piece of skin torn loose and hanging from the body. An amputation is the cutting or tearing off of a body part. Avulsions and amputations, while rare, can occur and should be handled like most other bleeding wounds. Be sure to use universal precautions to minimise the risk of infection. Call the ambulance service and control the bleeding and remember to care for both the exposed part and the avulsed or amputated part.

A nosebleed is bleeding from the nose. Nosebleeds occur more frequently in winter when allergies, respiratory infections, or dry air are associated with itching and picking of the nose. Blowing the nose too hard or hitting the nose can also cause nosebleeds.

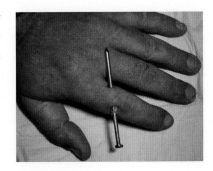

Figure 4-6

Puncture wound.

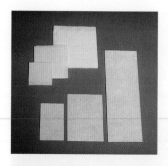

Figure 4-7

Dressings.

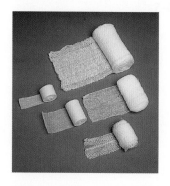

Figure 4-8

Bandages.

If a blood vessel breaks in the nostril, then blood runs out of the nostril. Tilting the child's head back or lying the child down may make the blood stop running out of the nostril, but it does not stop the bleeding. Some people mistakenly think they can stop a nosebleed by tipping the head back. You see less blood when the child lies down or tilts his head back because the blood drips down the back of the child's throat and the child swallows it. Swallowed blood upsets the stomach and may lead to vomiting. The stress of vomiting may make the nosebleed worse.

Open wounds may require dressings and bandages. A **dressing** is a clean covering placed over a wound (**Figure 4-7**). A **bandage** holds the dressing in place and also can be used to apply pressure to help control bleeding (**Figure 4-8**). **Plasters** are a combination of a dressing and a bandage. Commercial dressings, such as gauze pads, non-stick gauze pads, and adhesive bandages come in a variety of sizes. Sterile, commercially prepared, individually wrapped gauze pads are lint-free and easy to store in first aid supplies. Rolls of gauze can be used on any part of the body and come in various widths.

What You Should Look For

- Look carefully and see where the blood is coming from or where it seems to be accumulating under the skin. Children who have only a small cut under the top lip may have blood on their lips and tongue as well as on their shirts. Until you find the source of the blood, you might think that the lip, tongue, or face has been cut.
- Check if the blood is still flowing or if the flow has stopped.
- Observe whether the child who has had a big fall seems to be in pain or looks very ill. This may be a sign of internal bleeding.

What You Should Do

The Nine Steps in Paediatric First Aid:

1 Survey the Scene

Take a brief moment to perform a scene survey to ensure that the scene is safe, to find out who is involved, and to determine what happened.

2 Hands-off ABCs

As you approach the child, perform the hands-off ABCs (Appearance, Breathing, and Circulation) to determine if the ambulance service should be called. It should take 15 to 30 seconds or less.

3 Supervise

Immediately ensure that any other children near the scene are properly supervised.

4 Hands-on ABCDEs

Perform the hands-on ABCDEs (Appearance, Breathing, Circulation, Disability, and Everything else) to determine if the ambulance service should be called and what first aid care is needed.

5 First Aid Care

Provide first aid care appropriate to the injury or illness.

6 Notify

As soon as possible, notify the child's parent(s) or legal guardian(s).

7 Debrief

As soon as possible, talk with the child who received first aid about any concerns he or she may have, and talk with other children who witnessed the injury and first aid procedures.

8 Document

Complete an incident report form.

9 Prevention

Immediately remove or fence off any obvious danger. If this is not possible, report the hazard appropriately and place suitable signage up as an interim measure.

What You Should Do

First Aid Care for an Open Wound (Scrapes, Cuts, Tears, Avulsions, Amputations of Body Tissues)

 Follow Standard Precautions. Use a barrier between your skin and the bleeding wound. Protect your hand with a glove, a wad of towelling paper, or any other clean material that is available while you apply pressure to the wound.

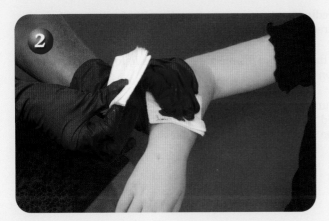

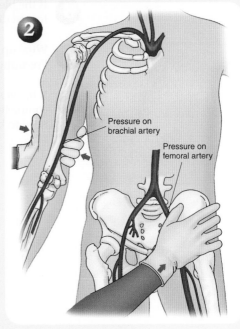

Pressure on brachial artery

Pressure on femoral artery

 Apply direct pressure with your fingers or the palm of your hand to the spot that is bleeding until the bleeding stops. Usually, bleeding will stop after 1 to 2 minutes of direct pressure. If you can control bleeding easily, wash the wound with soap and clean, running water, apply a bandage and follow up with the parent(s) or legal guardian(s). If bleeding is difficult to control, keep pressure on the wound for at least 5 minutes. If blood is seeping through the dressings while you apply pressure, do not remove the dressing that is in direct contact with the wound. Removing the dressing from contact with the wound may remove a clot that is forming to plug up the blood vessel that is bleeding. Apply additional dressings as needed. If the bleeding continues, apply pressure to one of the four pressure points. Pressure points are located in each of the upper arms and groin area of each leg. Applying pressure to these areas will slow the blood flow to the wound.

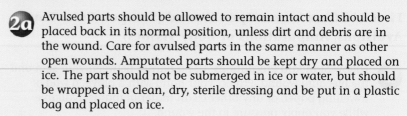

First Aid Care for an Open Wound (cont.)

2a Avulsed parts should be allowed to remain intact and should be placed back in its normal position, unless dirt and debris are in the wound. Care for avulsed parts in the same manner as other open wounds. Amputated parts should be kept dry and placed on ice. The part should not be submerged in ice or water, but should be wrapped in a clean, dry, sterile dressing and be put in a plastic bag and placed on ice.

3 If the bleeding continues or starts again after 5 minutes of sustained direct pressure, call the ambulance service.

4 Wipe up the spill and disinfect the surfaces following Standard Precautions.

5 If the wound is very dirty or tetanus prone and the child had not completed their tetanus immunisation programme, the child will need to be seen by a health care professional.

First Aid Tip

- A wound should be evaluated by a medical professional if it will not stay closed by itself, or requires 5 minutes of sustained direct pressure to control bleeding. The wound may require gluing or stitches.
- The edges of cuts longer than 3 to 4 centimetres may gape. These need to be managed by a medical professional who will use stitches, tape, glue, or some other special way to keep the edges of the skin together while the wound heals. To prevent infection and get the best healing, stitches are applied as soon as possible—generally within 6 hours of the injury.
- Prompt and proper cleaning, followed by closing of an open wound, reduces the risk of infection, promotes healing, and decreases scarring.
- A child can suck on an ice lolly to apply cold and pressure to cuts on lips or under the tongue, or to injured teeth.

What You Should Do

First Aid Care for Blisters

1 Protect blisters with a bandage. The bandage will help keep the blister from popping for as long as possible while the injured tissues under the blister heal.

2 Recommend to the parent(s) or legal guardian(s) that they should arrange for blisters that are larger than the diameter of a golf ball to be evaluated by a medical professional.

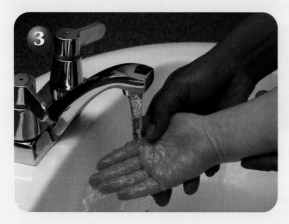

3 If the blister opens, clean it with water and care for it in the same way you treat an open wound.

What You Should Do

First Aid Care for Punctures, Including Splinters

1 With the child's parental consent, pull out small objects you can grasp easily, (e.g., a wood splinter or staple) with clean tweezers. If you cannot get a small object out easily, or if the object is large, or is deeply embedded, medical help is needed. Call the ambulance service if the penetrating object is large (e.g., a knife, stick, or an object embedded deeply below the skin). Do not pull out or move such an object. If appropriate, apply a bandage to keep the object from moving around or doing further damage.

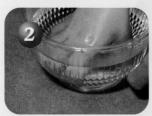

2 Soak the wound in clean water.

3 For wounds where the object has been removed, soak the wound again in clean water and then bandage the wound loosely or leave it without a bandage.

4 If the wound is considered to have a high risk of infection with tetanus spores and the child has not completed their full immunisation programme, the child will need to be seen by a health care professional as soon as possible.

What You Should Do

First Aid Care for Nosebleeds

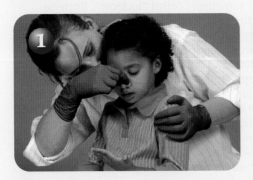
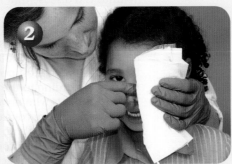

1 Keep the child sitting up.

2 Follow Standard Precautions. Use the thumb and a finger of one hand to pinch all of the soft parts of the nose together.

3 Position the child so that their head is tipped slightly forward. This stops blood running down the back of the throat.

4 Hold that position for a full 5 minutes. Do not peek to see if bleeding has stopped.

5 If you can, apply ice to the child's nose and cheeks using a plastic bag of ice or frozen vegetables wrapped in a cloth while you apply the pressure to the nose.

6 After 5 minutes of pressure, gently release the nose to avoid restarting the nosebleed. A sudden rush of blood re-entering the damaged blood vessel in the nose could dislodge the clot that formed while you kept the nose pinched and pressed against the face. If bleeding starts again, reapply the pressure, but for longer this time.

7 Have the child do a quiet activity for at least 30 minutes after the nosebleed stops, to avoid restarting the bleeding.

8 Avoid blowing the child's nose after stopping the nosebleed. Blowing the nose could dislodge the clot. If the child can do so easily, have the child blow out the excess blood right before you apply pressure so there will be less blood in the nose after the bleeding has been stopped. Since the blood forms scabs that can be itchy, large amounts of blood left in the nose may lead the child to pick and start the bleeding again.

9 Call the ambulance service or get medical help if a nosebleed cannot be controlled.

Did You Know

Tetanus is a disease that is sometimes called "lockjaw". Bacteria that cause tetanus live in the soil, dust, and in human and animal faeces. These bacteria enter the body through a dirty wound and the resulting tetanus causes strong spasms in the back, legs, arms, and jaw. The disease is often fatal, but routine tetanus vaccinations have made most people in the United Kingdom immune to tetanus. According to the latest guidance from the Department of Health, patients who have received a full course (five doses) of tetanus vaccine are considered to have lifelong immunity. Therefore, these individuals do not require a booster dose, even in the presence of a tetanus-prone wound. The primary course of three injections gives good protection for a number of years. The fourth and fifth doses ("boosters") maintain protection. After the fifth dose, immunity remains for life and you do not need any further boosters (apart from some travel situations).

Swelling

What You Should Know

With a **closed wound** the skin is not broken, but the tissue and blood vessels underneath the skin's surface are crushed, causing bleeding within a confined area. Closed wounds include **contusions** or bruises. Active children, especially those who engage in vigorous play, will often have bruises (**Figure 4-9**). Swelling can also occur with a closed wound.

Initially, a bruised area is red and swollen and then gradually turns blue or purple. As the blood is absorbed over the next few days, the area turns yellow and fades as it heals.

Figure 4-9

Bruise.

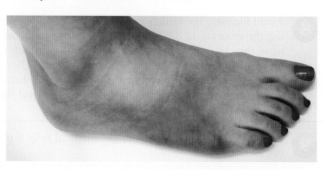

First Aid Tip

When a body part has been crushed, the damage may be more severe than is immediately apparent. Swelling from a crush injury can collapse the walls of blood vessels, pinching them and cutting off the necessary blood supply to tissues. If this condition continues, the tissues die. A medical professional must always evaluate crush injuries, even if they do not look severe.

What You Should Look For

- Check to see what caused the injury.
- Compare the injured part of the body with the same body part of the opposite side to see if there is swelling.
- Touch the skin to see if the skin feels tense.
- Look for discolouration of the skin over the injured area.
- If a body part was caught between two hard surfaces and squeezed or twisted, there may be a crush injury. If you have any suspicion that a crush injury occurred, proceed as if this is a potentially serious problem and arrange for the child to be evaluated by a medical professional.

What You Should Do

First Aid Care for Bruises and Swelling

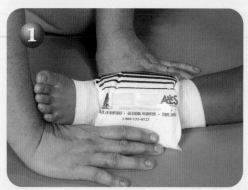

1 To control swelling, apply cold using ice, a bag of frozen vegetables, or a cold pack that is wrapped in a towel. Do not apply a frozen object directly against the skin because extreme cold may cause further injury. Care must also be taken in not leaving the ice pack on for too long, particularly in areas with thin muscle distribution. As a guide, the ice pack should be applied for between 5 and 15 minutes.

2 Call the ambulance service or get medical help if there is continued pain or swelling, or the child has had a crush injury.

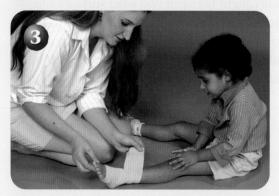

3 Stretchy rolled gauze or elastic bandages can be applied to put pressure on a bruised or a swollen area. They can also help to hold cold packs in place. If you use these bandages, leave the tips of fingers and toes exposed so that you can tell if the body part is wrapped too tightly. Check for changes in colour, temperature, and whether the fingers or toes lose their pink colour. The fingers or toes should have normal skin colour and feel warm to the touch.

4 Elevate the injury unless you suspect a broken bone or a spinal injury. Moving a child with a broken bone or a spinal injury can cause more injury to occur (see Musculoskeletal Injuries).

Algorithm

First Aid for Bleeding

Assess where blood is coming from
and whether the bleeding has stopped

Use a barrier between you and the blood, and
a plastic bag for contaminated articles

Apply direct pressure if bleeding is severe, otherwise flush
the wound with running water, and then apply direct
pressure to stop any bleeding

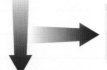

If the bleeding stops, apply a
dressing and bandage to the
wound

Call the ambulance service if
bleeding is severe or does not
stop within 5 minutes of
continuous direct pressure.
Continue to apply pressure until
ambulance personnel arrive,
without disturbing the dressing
that is touching the wound. Also
apply pressure to one of the four
pressure points. If all other
techniques fail, apply a
tourniquet to the affected limb,
above the wound.

Check Your Knowledge

1. To reduce the risk of infection, clean small wounds by:

a. Rubbing the dirt out with a soapy wash cloth.

b. Pouring alcohol on the injured area.

c. Flushing the injured area with running water.

d. Wiping the wound with a commercially packaged anti-septic wipe.

2. To control swelling in an injured part:

a. Put ice directly on the injury.

b. Place warm compresses on the injured body part.

c. Apply cold, wrap, and elevate the injured body part.

d. Place the injured part in a splint.

3. Describe all of the steps involved with treating a child who is bleeding severely.

_____

_____

_____

4. How would you treat a child with a nosebleed?

_____

_____

_____

Terms

Abrasions	Open wounds that occur when the top layer of skin is removed, with little blood loss.
Arteries	Large, deep, and well-protected blood vessels. Arteries carry blood under high pressure away from the heart to all parts of the body.
Bandage	Holds the dressing in place and also can be used to apply pressure to help control bleeding.
Blister	A collection of fluid in a bubble underneath the skin.
Capillaries	Tiny blood vessels located throughout the body which connect arteries to veins.
Closed wound	Type of wound where the skin is not broken, but the tissue and blood vessels underneath the skin's surface are crushed, causing bleeding within a confined area.
Contusion	An injury caused by a blow to the body that does not break the skin. Identified by swelling, discolouration, and pain.
Direct pressure	Applying pressure to a wound with your hand or with a firmly applied dressing.
Dressing	A clean covering placed over a wound.

Incision	A cut or break in the skin caused by something with a sharp edge such as a knife, razor blade, or glass. The edges of the wound look neat and will close together easily.
Internal bleeding	Injuries that occur deep in the chest, abdomen, or in the brain may be associated with bleeding in tissues far below the skin.
Laceration	A jagged break in the skin caused by tearing or blunt force. It will look more ragged than an incised wound.
Open wound	An injury that breaks the skin.
Plaster	A small piece of dressing held in place by a sticky bandage, usually only a few centimetres long
Puncture	A small hole made in the skin, which may be either deep or shallow.
Standard Precautions	Measures required to protect against contact with any body fluids that might contain blood. Precautions include cleaning and disinfecting surfaces that have come in contact with any type of body fluids (except sweat) and hand washing.
Tourniquet	A lifesaving device used to control severe bleeding consisting of a constricting band placed around a limb tightly, causing the blood to stop flowing into the limb and thus out of a wound.

| **Universal Precautions** | Protective measures that apply to blood, bodily fluids that might contain blood, and sexual secretions. They do not apply to faeces, nasal secretions, sputum, sweat, tears, urine, and vomitus. |
| **Veins** | Blood vessels that carry blood back to the heart. |

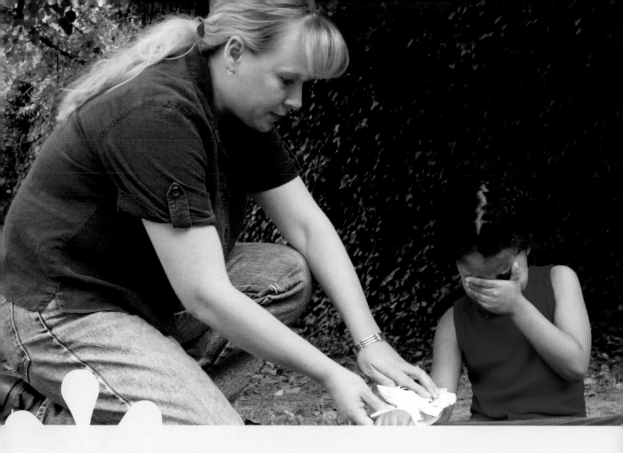

Learning Objectives

The participant will be able to:

- Define closed and open fracture.
- Describe how to use DOTS (Deformity, Open injury, Tenderness, and Swelling) to assess a musculoskeletal injury.
- Describe how to use RICE (Rest, Ice, Compression, Elevation) to treat a minor musculoskeletal injury.
- Identify the appropriate response to suspected:
  a. Broken bones (fractures)
  b. Dislocations
  c. Sprains
  d. Injuries to the spine

Chapter 5

Bone, Joint, and Muscle Injuries

Bone, Joint, and Muscle Injuries

Introduction

The bones and joints of young children are generally more flexible than those of adults. Unlike adults, children rarely strain or tear muscles and ligaments while stretching, bending, or running. However, young children are more prone to dislocation of the joints than adults, especially dislocation of the elbow. Due to their impulsive behaviour, children frequently experience broken bones and bruises. Spinal injuries involve the bones and joints of the spine, muscles that surround the spine, or the spinal cord and nerves. Collectively, bones, joints, and muscles are called the **musculoskeletal system**.

What You Should Know

A **fracture** is a broken bone. Any bone in the body can be fractured, including those of the limbs, trunk, and spine. A fracture can be a partial break or a complete break in the bone. The surrounding muscles, nerves, and blood vessels can also be damaged when the bone is fractured.

Fractures are common in children. Fortunately, children's bones heal more rapidly after a fracture than those of adults. Although healing is usually complete, sometimes a fracture can cause trouble with growth or full range of motion in the part of the body where the bone was broken.

A **closed fracture** occurs when the skin is not broken at the location of the fracture. An **open fracture** occurs when there is an open wound over the fracture. The wound can occur either from the broken edge of the bone cutting through the tissues and skin, or from the force that broke the bone (**Figure 5-1**). The event of blood loss is equal in open and closed fractures, but the blood loss is more obvious in open fractures and there is a greater chance of infection.

A **dislocation** is the separation of a bone from a joint. In children, dislocations commonly happen to fingers and elbows, and are

Figure 5-1

Closed fracture (A), open fracture (B).

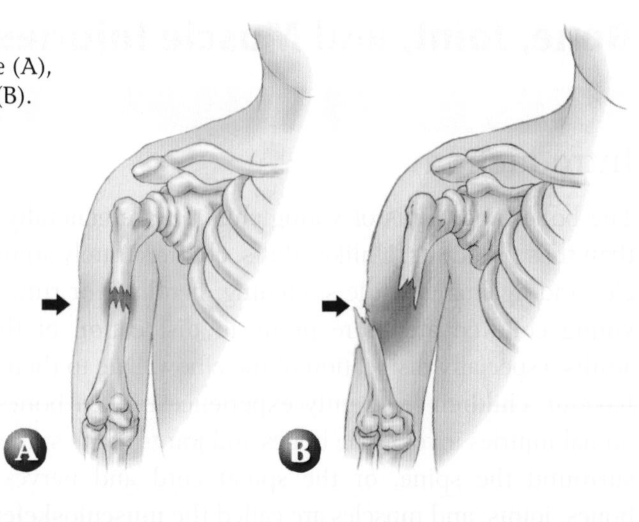

not always obvious. It takes only a small amount of force to dislocate a child's bone. A quick tug on a child's hand to prevent the child from stepping into the street or to protect against a stumble can be enough to dislocate an elbow. Infants and young children should not be picked up by their hands or wrists (**Figure 5-2**).

Sometimes a dislocated bone will go back into the socket by itself right away, but often a medical professional will need to return the bone to its proper position. Loss of movement of the joint causes pain if the bone remains dislocated.

A **sprain** is an injury that occurs when the tissues that hold the joints together (**ligaments**) are stretched beyond their limits. A **strain** occurs when a force stretches a muscle or muscles beyond their limits. Sprains are uncommon in young children but begin to occur in children as they progress through secondary school, and their joints become more like adult joints.

At the time of the injury, most children do not want to move a body part that has a fractured bone or a significantly hurt muscle or joint. The injury causes pain and muscle spasm and generally makes children hold the injured body part still. Children may "splint" their own injured body part by holding it against their body or by just holding the body part very still.

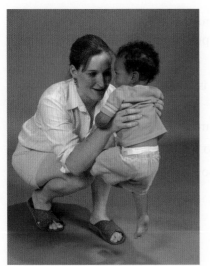

Figure 5-2

Lift children under their arms, not by hands or wrists.

It is not necessary for someone giving first aid to figure out whether there is a fracture, dislocation, sprain, or strain. First aid is the same for any of these injuries. The role of the person giving first aid is to recognise that the child has a potentially serious injury and then use techniques that keep the injured part from moving until a medical professional can evaluate the injury.

First Aid Tip

Do not worry if you are unable to figure out whether the injury is a fracture, dislocation, strain, or sprain as the treatment is similar for any of these injuries.

What You Should Look For

You should suspect a child may have a musculoskeletal injury based on your initial survey of the scene. If a child has fallen or been struck by some force, some injury to muscles, bones, or joints might have occurred. As you approach the child and are doing your hands-off ABCs, you can observe whether the child is in pain or seems to be holding some body part still in an unnatural way. If a bone, joint, or muscle injury has occurred, the child will complain of pain at the injury site. Even if the child is crying, you can try to get the child to point to where it hurts. Asking the child to point to the spot that hurts helps distract the child from the intensity of the pain and helps you avoid jumping to a wrong conclusion about what body part has been hurt. It can be hard to figure out where the injury is located when you see the child crying or refusing to move. The child may be holding an uninjured part to keep the injured part still. Children figure out within seconds that avoiding movement of an injured part reduces the pain.

When dealing with bone, joint, and muscle injuries, use the mnemonic **DOTS (Deformity, Open injury, Tenderness, Swelling)** to assess the extent of the injury.

- Deformity is when a bone is broken and causes an abnormal shape.
- Open injuries or wounds are a break in the skin.
- Tenderness is sensitivity to touch.
- Swelling is the body's response to injury that makes the area look larger than usual.

When muscles, bones, or joints are injured, blood and other fluids collect around the injury. This accumulation of fluid causes swelling. Sometimes a break in the bone results in an unnatural shape or bend of the body part. This unnatural appearance is called a deformity. You can recognise a deformity from your assessment of appearance when you do the hands-off ABCs and hands-on ABCDEs. To detect a deformity, compare the injured body part with the uninjured side. Remember that loss of movement tells you that a bone, muscle, or joint injury may have occurred. The child may be able to move the injured part slightly, but not have full range of motion. In the hands-on ABCDEs, this loss of function is the "D" for disability.

What You Should Do

The Nine Steps in Paediatric First Aid:

1) Survey the Scene

Take a brief moment to perform a scene survey to ensure that the scene is safe, to find out who is involved, and to determine what happened.

2) Hands-off ABCs

As you approach the child, perform the hands-off ABCs (Appearance, Breathing, and Circulation) to determine if the ambulance service should be called. It should take 15 to 30 seconds or less.

3) Supervise

Immediately ensure that any other children near the scene are properly supervised.

4) Hands-on ABCDEs

Perform the hands-on ABCDEs (Appearance, Breathing, Circulation, Disability, and Everything else) to determine if the ambulance service should be called and what first aid care is needed.

5 First Aid Care
Provide first aid care appropriate to the injury or illness.

6 Notify
As soon as possible, notify the child's parent(s) or legal guardian(s).

7 Debrief
As soon as possible, talk with the child who received first aid about any concerns he or she may have, and talk with other children who witnessed the injury and first aid procedures.

8 Document
Complete an incident report form.

9 Prevention
Immediately remove or fence off any obvious danger. If this is not possible, report the hazard appropriately and place suitable signage up as an interim measure.

What You Should Do

First Aid for Bone, Joint, and Muscle Injuries

First aid and subsequent care for musculoskeletal injuries are known by the mnemonic **RICE (Rest, Ice, Compression, and Elevation)**. If the child can move the body part and it only hurts a little bit, the injury is often minor. Otherwise, a medical professional should evaluate the injury to decide what care is appropriate. Minor injuries can be managed with the measures indicated by RICE.

1. Rest. Have the child assume a comfortable position (e.g., sitting or lying down). Pain is the body's way of indicating that a problem exists. If movement of an injured body part is painful, the child should not be urged to move it. However,

unless otherwise advised, it is important to encourage the child to mobilise an injured limb to promote good blood flow and tissue repair, this also improves the recovery time.

2. Ice. Cover the injury with a cloth and apply ice or a cold pack for periods of 5 to 15 minutes every 2 hours for the first 24 to 48 hours. This reduces pain, bleeding, and swelling. Having a cloth between the ice and the skin protects the skin from extreme cold. An elastic bandage is a good way to hold the ice or cold pack in place. Continuous use of ice or direct contact of ice with the skin can damage the tissue (**Figure 5-3A**).

3. Compression. You can use an elastic bandage to compress the injured area. This limits the collection of blood and other fluids. Start a few centimetres below and end several centimetres above the injury. Wrap upward toward the heart in a spiral manner. Use firm, even pressure, making sure you do not wrap too tightly. If the child complains that the fingers or toes are cold, tingling, or becoming numb, loosen the bandage. Remove the elastic bandage only when applying ice (**Figure 5-3B**).

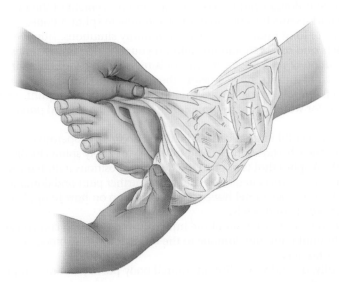

Figure 5-3A

RICE. A. Ice.

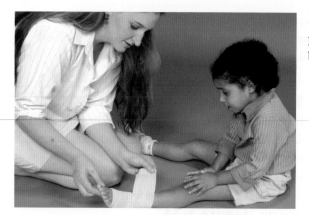

Figure 5-3B
RICE.
B. Compression.

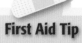

First Aid Tip

- Do not wrap a compression bandage too tightly.
- Assess the colour of the area below the bandage to assure that the bandage is not too tight.
- Always protect the skin by wrapping the ice in a thin cloth.
- Do not use ice for longer than 5 to 15 minutes at a time because it can damage the tissue.

4. Elevation. Elevate the injury above the level of the heart by placing the injured limb on several pillows. This limits blood flow to the injury and reduces swelling.

Did You Know

Splinting in a Child Care Setting

Splinting is doing what is necessary to limit movement of the injured part as much as possible. Knowing how to splint a bone, muscle, or joint injury can be useful in many situations. However, teachers and carers should not splint a young child's injury unless application of pressure on the injury is required to control bleeding or the child must be moved before the ambulance can arrive. Instead, ambulance personnel should apply any needed splint. The reasons for waiting for the ambulance to splint the injured parts are:

- A young child in pain cannot be relied on to be cooperative.
- Someone who has only first aid training can apply splints incorrectly. A splint that is applied too tightly or positions a limb incorrectly can restrict circulation and cause further pain and damage.
- Ambulance personnel have received training on how to apply a splint easily and safely.
- Unnecessary movement of the injury during splinting can cause additional pain and damage to the bone, soft tissue, blood vessels, and nerves.
- Usually, a child will splint an injured body part by not moving it to avoid pain.

First Aid Tip

Splinting
It is generally better to wait for the ambulance service to arrive to splint an injured body part. You may need to splint the injured body part to control bleeding or if you must move the child. To splint an injured body part, you can:
- Put it against an uninjured part of the child's body. For example, you can tape an injured finger to an uninjured finger next to it (commonly called "buddy-strapping").
- Use a rigid object that is big enough to cross the joint above and below the injury. Put the rigid object against the injured body part and use cloth or tape to hold it in place. This helps to prevent the broken bone edges from moving.

If a wound is present follow Standard Precautions. To control bleeding when there may be a bone injury, apply pressure on the tissues above or below the injury or directly on any bone end that is bleeding. Be sure that the ends of the broken bone do not move during the application of pressure to control bleeding. If the bone ends move, further injury might occur. If you need to control bleeding, **splinting** the injured area may help to prevent movement at the site of the injury.

After controlling bleeding, cover the wound with a sterile dressing or a large, clean cloth to keep the injured area as clean as possible.

Apply ice or cold packs wrapped in a thin towel to reduce swelling and pain. Elevate a splinted injured arm or leg, as long as it does not cause increased pain. This also helps to reduce swelling and pain. Do not move anyone you suspect might have a neck or spinal injury.

First Aid Tip

- Do not attempt to clean an open wound if you suspect that there is a fracture.
- Do not give the child who might have a broken bone anything to eat or drink.
- Do not move anyone you suspect might have a neck or spinal injury.

Injuries to the Spine

What Should You Know

The spine is comprised of 33 bones (or **vertebrae**) that provide a framework to keep the body upright. Most vertebra have a whole in the middle, and when all lined up, these holes create a tube in which the **spinal cord** is located. The spinal cord is attached to the bottom of the brain and conveys messages from the brain to the body via lots of nerves that originate along its length. A **spinal injury** may occur to the vertebrae, the cord, or the nerves and the effects of an injury to any of these parts may be severe. Any serious injury can cause **paralysis** below the area of injury. Paralysis is a permanent loss of feeling and movement.

Fractures of the spine are uncommon in children. However, any child who is unresponsive after an event that could have caused a spinal injury should be treated as if he has a spinal injury (**Figure 5-4**). If a child with a spinal injury is allowed to sit up or is improperly handled, nerves can become damaged which can cause paralysis and death.

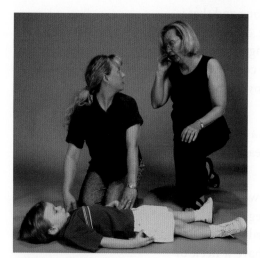

Figure 5-4

Keep a child with a suspected back or neck (spinal) injury still. A child who is unresponsive after an injury should be treated as if there may be a spinal injury.

What You Should Look For

- Loss of responsiveness.
- Child is unable to walk or experiences muscle spasms.
- Neck or back pain.
- Localised tenderness, swelling, or bruising.
- Headaches—child complains of pain radiating through shoulders.
- Child is unable to move arms or legs.
- Loss of mobility—child will not want to move the neck.

What You Should Do

First Aid Care for Spinal Injuries

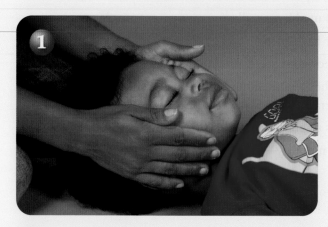

1 Ensure that the child does not move and that nobody moves him. Do not struggle with the child or hold him down. A child with a spine injury will either be unable to move or will find that moving hurts and will not want to move.

2 Call the ambulance service to transport the child to a medical facility.

Algorithm

First Aid for Bone, Joint, and Muscle Injuries

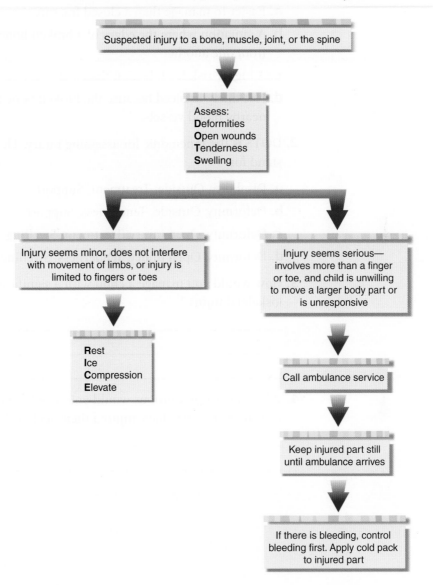

Suspected injury to a bone, muscle, joint, or the spine

Assess:
Deformities
Open wounds
Tenderness
Swelling

Injury seems minor, does not interfere with movement of limbs, or injury is limited to fingers or toes

Injury seems serious— involves more than a finger or toe, and child is unwilling to move a larger body part or is unresponsive

Rest
Ice
Compression
Elevate

Call ambulance service

Keep injured part still until ambulance arrives

If there is bleeding, control bleeding first. Apply cold pack to injured part

Check Your Knowledge

1. An open fracture is:

   a. Easier to manage than a closed fracture.

   b. A situation where the edges of a broken bone separate from one another.

   c. A bigger risk for infection than a closed fracture.

   d. Not likely to bleed because the broken bone presses on nearby blood vessels.

2. DOTS is the mnemonic for assessing injury. The letters stand for:

   a. Disability, Outside, Treatment, Support.

   b. Deformity, Outside, Tenderness, Support.

   c. Deformity, Open injury, Treatment, Swelling.

   d. Deformity, Open injury, Tenderness, Swelling.

3. How would you manage a child with a significant musculoskeletal injury?

_____

_____

_____

4. What special precautions would you take for a child who you suspected may have injured their neck or back?

_____

_____

_____

Terms

Closed fracture	When the skin is not broken where the bone is fractured.
Dislocation	The separation of a bone from a joint.
DOTS	Mnemonic for assessing injury to the musculoskeletal system: Deformity, Open injury, Tenderness, Swelling.
Fracture	A broken bone.
Ligaments	The tissues that hold the joints together.
Musculoskeletal system	Bones, joints and muscles, collectively.
Open fracture	When there is an open wound over the fracture caused either by the bone breaking through the skin or by the skin being torn by the force of whatever caused the break in the bone.
Paralysis	A permanent loss of feeling and movement.
RICE	Mnemonic for first aid care for a musculoskeletal injury: Rest, Ice, Compression, Elevation.
Spinal cord	Nerve tissue that is found in the bony column (spine) and connects the brain to the body via smaller nerves that originate along its length.
Spinal injury	An injury that damages the spinal cord, nerves or vertebrae.
Splinting	Holding an injured body part still.
Sprain	Occurs when ligaments are stretched beyond their limits.
Strain	An injury that occurs when a force stretches a muscle or muscles beyond their limits.
Vertebrae	Thirty-three bones that are stacked on each other forming a spinal column.

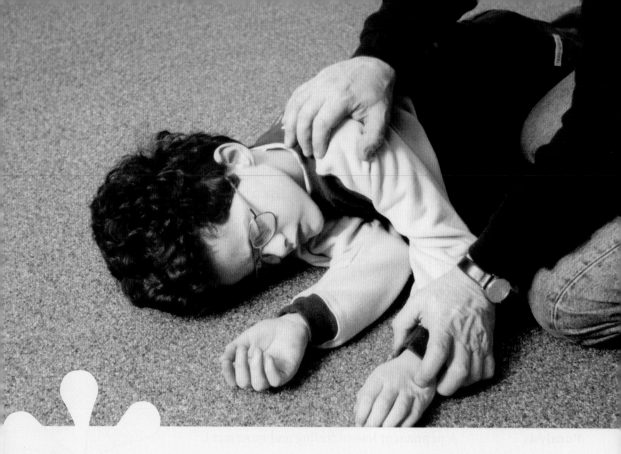

Learning Objectives

The participant will be able to:

- Recognise the causes, signs, and symptoms of fainting.
- Describe first aid for fainting.
- Identify some causes of loss of consciousness.
- Identify the difference between hypoglycaemia and hyperglycaemia.
- Identify some risk factors for head injuries in childhood.
- Describe signs and symptoms of a concussion.
- Identify signs of an internal head injury that would indicate a child needs immediate care by a medical professional.
- Describe first aid for a head injury.

Chapter

6

Loss of Consciousness, Fainting, and Head Injuries

Loss of Consciousness, Fainting, and Head Injuries

Introduction

Loss of consciousness can occur for multiple reasons. Injury, low blood sugar, stress, severe allergic reactions, and even breath holding may be associated with loss of consciousness in children. Fainting is a loss of consciousness that is not caused by injury. Children can suffer head injuries as a result of fainting.

Head injuries are common during childhood years. For every 100,000 children under 5 years of age, 82 will suffer a traumatic injury each year. Most of these injuries are caused by falls. The relative heaviness of a toddler's head makes head injuries more common (**Figure 6-1**). After falls, the second most common cause of head injury is motor vehicle crashes.

Most head injuries do not injure the brain, but may leave superficial bruising and/or swelling of the skin, or a "**goose egg**". The size of a bump on the head does not correlate with the severity of the head injury.

The main concern with a head injury is bleeding or swelling inside the skull. This can occur even when the skull itself does not appear to be damaged. Some internal head injuries can be severe enough to cause permanent brain damage or even death.

First Aid Tip

The size of any lump or bump on the head does not correlate with the severity of the child's head injury.

Figure 6-1

The relative heaviness of a toddler's head makes head injuries more common.

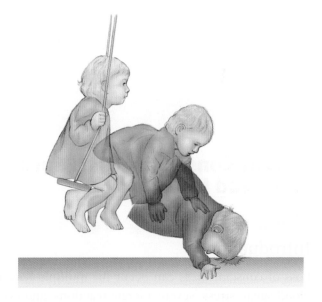

Fainting

What You Should Know

Fainting is a sudden and temporary loss of responsiveness caused by a brief lack of blood and oxygen to the brain. Fainting is not caused by an injury; it is a nervous system reaction to such situations as fear, pain, or strong emotional upset. Occasionally, prolonged standing in a warm environment results in fainting. Typically, fainting is not serious. Usually, children recover from the event in a few minutes without any special care.

Either lowering the head below the heart or raising the feet above the level of the heart can prevent fainting by allowing more blood to flow to the brain. Some children who faint assume an unusual posture while they are unresponsive. These individuals may bend their hands at the wrist and stiffen their legs. Unlike a seizure, there are no jerking movements.

What You Should Look For

- Lightheadedness
- Dizziness
- Nausea
- Pale skin colour
- Sweating

What You Should Do

The Nine Steps in Paediatric First Aid:

1 Survey the Scene

Take a brief moment to perform a scene survey to ensure that the scene is safe, to find out who is involved, and to determine what happened.

2 Hands-off ABCs

As you approach the child, perform the hands-off ABCs (Appearance, Breathing, and Circulation) to determine if the ambulance service should be called. It should take 15 to 30 seconds or less.

3 Supervise

Immediately ensure that any other children near the scene are properly supervised.

4 Hands-on ABCDEs

Perform the hands-on ABCDEs (Appearance, Breathing, Circulation, Disability, and Everything else) to determine if the ambulance service should be called and what first aid care is needed.

5 First Aid Care

Provide first aid care appropriate to the injury or illness.

6 Notify

As soon as possible, notify the child's parent(s) or legal guardian(s).

7 Debrief

As soon as possible, talk with the child who received first aid about any concerns he or she may have, and talk with other children who witnessed the injury and first aid procedures.

8 Document

Complete an incident report form.

9 Prevention

Immediately remove or fence off any obvious danger. If this is not possible, report the hazard appropriately and place suitable signage up as an interim measure.

What You Should Do

First Aid Care for Fainting

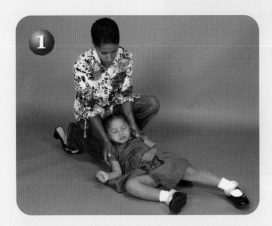

1 Lay the child on her back to prevent falling. If the child has already fainted, position the child on her back and check for breathing. If the child is not breathing, follow the steps outlined on page 36.

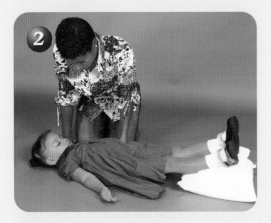

2 Elevate the legs 20 to 30 centimetres to increase blood flow to the brain.

3 Loosen tight-fitting clothing.

First Aid Care for Fainting (cont.)

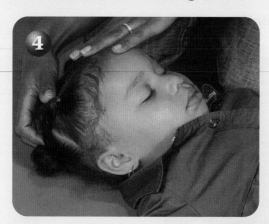

4 Call the ambulance service if the child remains unresponsive for more than a minute or so after positioning her with her legs elevated.

5 Look for a potential cause for the loss of consciousness. Consider the following possibilities:

- Injury
- Blood loss
- Ingestion of a medicine or poison
- Allergic reaction
- Extreme temperatures
- Fatigue
- Illness
- Stress
- Not eating
- Standing still for long periods
- A breath-holding spell

6 Record details of the event. This includes the amount of time the child was unconscious, possible cause, symptoms and signs (e.g., nausea, vomiting, decreased level of alertness, unresponsiveness, perspiration), nature of any fall, and duration of each symptom.

7 Inform the parent(s) or legal guardian(s) that the child has fainted, as this child may need to be seen by a health care professional.

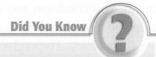

Did You Know

Breath-Holding Spells
Some young children cause themselves to faint by holding their breath. In a young child, frustration, anger, and fear can sometimes lead to breath holding. Often, uncontrolled crying occurs before breath holding. As with other types of fainting, children will lose responsiveness for 20 to 45 seconds. Children begin to breathe normally after fainting and then regain responsiveness. There is no specific treatment other than usual care for fainting. Teachers, carers, and parent(s) or legal guardian(s) may attempt to teach the child to manage their feelings to reduce the episodes. However, the problem often disappears as the child matures and learns better coping skills.

Diabetes

What You Should Know

Diabetes is a medical condition which affects millions of people throughout the world. It is a condition in which the body cannot regulate the sugars in the blood stream. This inability to regulate sugar is due to the body's inability to produce insulin or react to insulin.

There are two (2) types of diabetes:

- Type 1 – (previously called "Juvenile Onset Diabetes") Children with Type 1 diabetes do not produce enough insulin to regulate the sugars in the body. These children must take insulin either by injection or through an insulin pump.
- Type II – (previously called "Adult Onset") Type II is the most common form of diabetes. This type is caused by either the body's inability to produce enough insulin or the body is not reacting to it adequately.

It is important to know the difference between hypoglycaemia and hyperglycaemia when talking about diabetes. **Hypoglycaemia** is a condition in which the body does not have enough sugar. Without sugar, the body cannot work effectively as sugar is needed for energy. This condition may occur when the child does not eat enough, takes too much insulin, exercises too much, is overheated, or possibly due to an illness. **Hyperglycaemia** is the opposite of hypoglycaemia. It occurs when the body has too much sugar in the blood. This condition may be caused by insufficient insulin, overeating, inactivity, illness, stress, or a combination of these factors.

What You Should Look For

Signs of hypoglycaemia include:

- Slurred speech
- Drowsiness
- Paleness
- Confusion
- Trembling
- Staggering
- Poor coordination
- Irritability
- Excessive sweating
- Eventual unconsciousness

Signs of hyperglycaemia include:

- Extreme thirst
- Drowsiness
- Fruit smell on child's breath
- Rapid breathing
- Warm, dry skin
- Very frequent urination
- Vomiting
- Eventual unconsciousness

What You Should Do

For hypoglycaemia, treatment includes giving sugar (granular by tea-spoon on the tongue or under the tongue or by drinking orange juice). If the child does not begin to act normally, call the ambulance service and give more sugar. For hyperglycaemia, treatment includes calling the ambulance service. If you are unsure which condition the child may be experiencing, either hypoglycaemia or hyperglycaemia, it is acceptable to give sugar and determine whether or not that helps if the child is awake and aware.

Head Injuries

What You Should Know

Head injuries commonly affect the scalp. The scalp has many blood vessels and even small cuts can cause a lot of bleeding. Swelling can take on the appearance of a goose egg after an injury. These areas of swelling can take days or weeks to heal.

Internal head injury refers to damage to the brain. When the head receives a forceful blow, the brain strikes the inside of the skull, resulting in some degree of injury. In addition, blood and other flu-ids can accumulate inside the skull, placing pressure on the brain.

Did You Know ?

Young infants have openings in the skull, called **fontanelles.** These areas are commonly known as "soft spots" (**Figure 6-2**). Al-though the skull bone has not yet formed, a very tough covering of tissue protects the brain under the soft spots. Injury to the brain in the area of the fontanelles is rare, but bulging of the soft spots indi-cates abnormal pressure in the skull. A sunken fontanelle can indi-cate dehydration. The back (posterior) fontanelle closes around 2 months after birth and the front (anterior) fontanelle closes around 18 to 24 months.

Figure 6-2

Fontanelles.

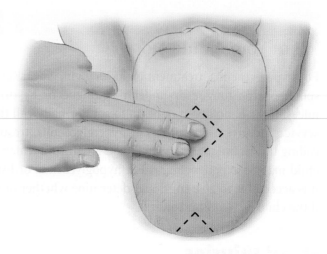

Concussion is a term that generally refers to the symptoms of dizziness and nausea, with or without a loss of consciousness, after a violent jarring of the brain.

What You Should Look For

- Bleeding from any part of the head
- Loss of consciousness. Appearing stunned for several seconds after a head injury is not the same as being unconscious. Unconsciousness can last for just a few seconds or for as long as several days. Crying immediately after the injury is a good sign.
- Signs of confusion or memory loss. A child should know where she is, and recall the event even if she is upset after the injury.
- Pale, sweaty appearance
- Severe headache
- Nausea or vomiting more than once
- Wetting pants or losing bowel control (when unusual for that child)
- Blurred vision
- Unusual sleepiness, listlessness, or tiring easily

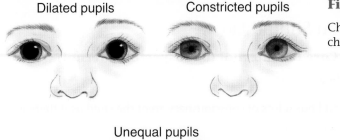

Dilated pupils   Constricted pupils

Figure 6-3

Check the child's pupils.

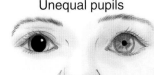

Unequal pupils

- Agitation, combativeness, irritability, crankiness
- Pupils of unequal size. Check how pupils constrict (get smaller) when exposed to light (**Figure 6-3**).
- Difficulty with walking, speech, or balance
- Seizure
- Swelling of an infant's fontanelle
- Fluid (blood or clear) dripping from the nose or ear
- Changes in eating patterns, sleeping patterns, or the way the child is playing or performing (for example, lack of interest in a favourite toy or activity)
- Loss of a new skill, such as speech, walking, or toilet training

First Aid Tip

Commonly, children vomit after banging their heads. One occurrence is not necessarily a sign to be alarmed about, particularly in the absence of any other signs or symptoms. Immediate medical assistance should be sought however, if the child continues to vomit or develops nausea.

Did You Know ❓

If the child vomits before regaining full consciousness, you should turn the child's entire body and head together to the left side. Rolling the child to the left side helps to reduce vomiting. Having the child rolled on the side helps avoid choking on the vomit. Rolling the child's entire body and head together (logroll) helps protect the child from the possibility that movement will worsen an injured neck or spine.

What You Should Do

First Aid Care for Internal (or Suspected Internal) Head Injury

1 If a child has a loss of consciousness, treat the child as if there is also a spine injury.

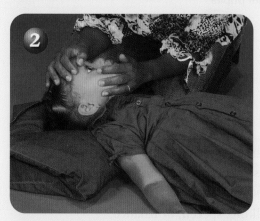

2 If the child is alert, look in the pupils. The pupils widen in darkness and narrow in brighter light. Look to see if the pupils are round, equal to one another, and about the same size as those of other people in the same light.

3 Contact the ambulance service if the child shows any signs or symptoms of internal head injury listed above or if the child lost consciousness.

4 If there are no problems noted on the assessment, the child requires close observation for about 6 hours after the injury and then ongoing observation of any changed behaviour for the next few days. The parent(s) or legal guardian(s) should consult a medical professional and become informed about how to watch for signs and symptoms of a head injury and create a plan of action if abnormalities develop.

What You Should Do

First Aid for an Open Head Injury

1 Follow Standard Precautions.

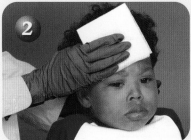

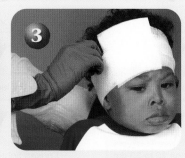

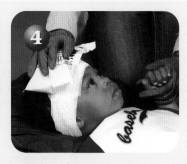

2 Apply gentle pressure to control any bleeding. Gentle pressure is better than heavy pressure if the skull is fractured.

3 Put a clean bandage on the wound once bleeding has stopped. If the bleeding does not stop with continuous pressure, call the ambulance service.

4 Put a cool pack on the injured area for 10 to 15 minutes. (Wrap ice or a frozen object that you are using as a cold pack in a thin cloth so that direct contact with skin does not cause injury.)

First Aid Tip

Sleeping After a Head Injury
- Allow the child to sleep if there are no other signs or symptoms of internal head injury and if it is a normal bed or naptime.
- If the child is acting normally before the regularly scheduled bed or naptime, allow the child to sleep for up to 2 hours without being awakened. After 2 hours of sleeping, when awakening the child, check to see if the child wakes up as easily as usual. Get medical help if the child is not acting normally.
- Note that sleep does not worsen a head injury. The concern is that a sleeping child cannot be observed for changes in behaviour or level of consciousness.

Algorithm

First Aid for Fainting

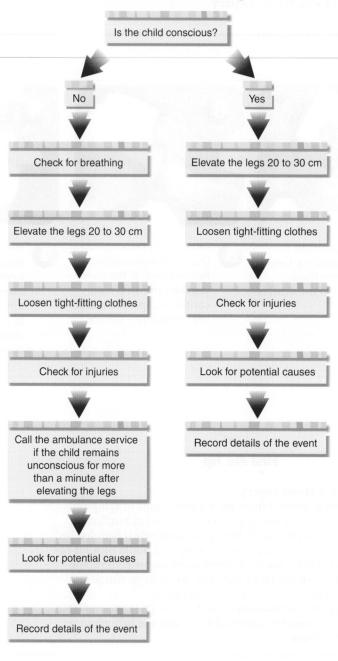

First Aid for Internal Head Injury

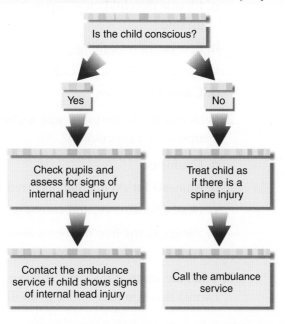

First Aid for Open Head Injuries

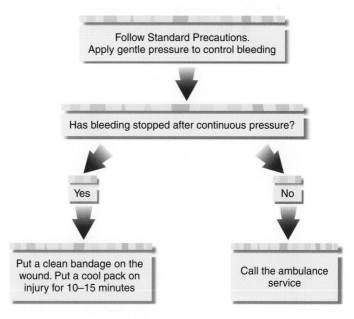

Check Your Knowledge

1. Which of the following is not correct first aid for fainting?

    a. Elevate the child's legs, up to 30 centimetres off the ground

    b. Loosen tight clothing

    c. Put a cold pack on the child's face

    d. Check for injuries

2. Which of the following would *not* be considered a sign or symptom of a concussion?

    a. Confusion

    b. Amnesia for events that occurred after the head injury

    c. Headache, nausea, and vomiting multiple times

    d. Silence in the first moments after a fall, followed by crying

3. What are some of the signs and symptoms of hypoglycaemia that you may notice in an ill child?

_____

_____

_____

4. What are the signs and symptoms of a child suffering from concussion?

_____

_____

_____

Terms

Concussion	Generally refers to the symptoms of dizziness and nausea, with or without loss of consciousness, after a violent jarring of the brain.
Diabetes	A disease in which the body is unable to regulate sugar normally because of a deficiency or lack of insulin or an inability to react to insulin.
Fainting	A sudden and temporary loss of consciousness caused by a brief lack of blood and oxygen to the brain.
Fontanelles	Openings in the skull found in young infants, often called soft spots.
Goose egg	Superficial bruising and/or swelling of the skin on the head.
Hyperglycaemia	Abnormally high blood sugar level.
Hypoglycaemia	Abnormally low blood sugar level.
Internal head injury	Damage to the brain. When the head receives a forceful blow, the brain strikes the inside of the skull, resulting in some degree of injury.

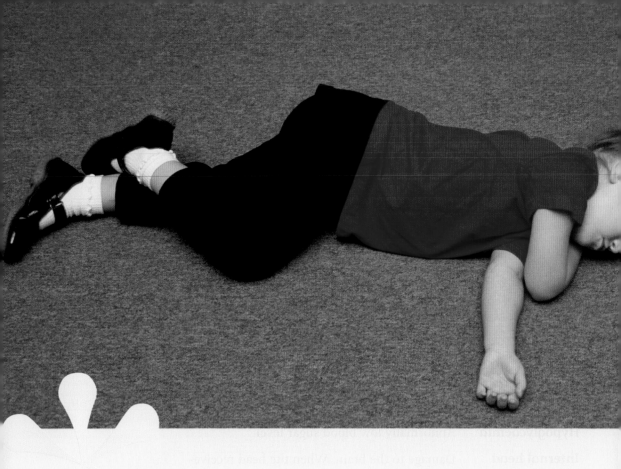

Learning Objectives

The participant will be able to:

- Recognise convulsive and non-convulsive seizures.
- Identify appropriate first aid for convulsive or non-convulsive seizures.

Chapter

7

Convulsions and Seizures

Seizures

Introduction

Seizures are caused by a disturbance in the electrical impulses of the brain. These disturbances result in a variety of body responses. These range from the very mild, such as a few moments of staring, to the more severe, such as loss of consciousness and convulsions.

A seizure can be convulsive or non-convulsive. **Convulsive seizures** are characterised by involuntary muscle contractions and body movement. **Non-convulsive seizures** are associated with confusion and loss of awareness.

What You Should Know

A variety of conditions can cause a seizure, including: an inherited disorder, high fever, head injury, serious illness, or poisoning. A child who experiences a seizure for the first time should always receive immediate emergency medical care.

Sometimes a specific cause of the seizure can be identified. More commonly, however, the cause remains unknown. Even without knowing the exact cause, a medical professional can usually treat the child with medication to control the seizures or reduce their frequency.

The most easily recognisable seizure involves the entire body and is called a **tonic-clonic seizure** (previously called grand mal). When a seizure is about to happen, an older child might know that the seizure is coming by recognizing a brief feeling or sensation that comes on just prior to the beginning of the seizure, known as an **aura.** This is somewhat of an internal warning system, which can be a noise, visual change, funny taste, numbness, or another feeling. Some children experience no aura or do not recognise it so they do not know that the seizure is about to start.

Partial seizures (previously called petit mal), or absences occur when consciousness is affected and the child may lose their sense of awareness and have no memory of the event. The child may stare off into space or make an unusual noise or expression, and then return to what they were doing with no recollection of the last few seconds.

A **febrile convulsion** is a seizure caused by a rapid rise in body temperature. The body temperature does not have to be very high, but the rate of change in body temperature is fast. In a small percentage of children, a rapid rise in fever can cause a convulsion. A febrile convulsion is not related to a life-long convulsion disorder. This type of convulsion usually has no effect on the child's nervous system, development, or brain function. Febrile convulsions occur most frequently between 6 months and 6 years of age. A child who has experienced a febrile convulsion is more likely to have another one than a child who has never had one. Febrile convulsions usually stop in a few minutes, without any special care. A convulsion that lasts more than 5 minutes is not likely to be a febrile in origin, and the ambulance service should be contacted.

A child who has a febrile convulsion for the first time should be seen by a medical professional as soon as possible. If the child has experienced a febrile convulsion, the parent(s) or legal guardian(s) should speak with the child's medical professional to get instructions for how to handle the situation, if it happens again.

What You Should Look For

The signs and symptoms of seizure include one or more of the following:

- Loss of consciousness or responsiveness
- Breathing that stops temporarily
- Rigid body with jerking and shaking movements of the entire body
- Neck and back arching
- Eyes rolling back
- Increased saliva production, causing drooling or foaming at the mouth
- Loss of control of bladder or bowels

What You Should Do

The Nine Steps in Paediatric First Aid:

1 Survey the Scene

Take a brief moment to perform a scene survey to ensure that the scene is safe, to find out who is involved, and to determine what happened.

(2) Hands-off ABCs

As you approach the child, perform the hands-off ABCs (Appearance, Breathing, and Circulation) to determine if the ambulance service should be called. It should take 15 to 30 seconds or less.

(3) Supervise

Immediately ensure that any other children near the scene are properly supervised.

(4) Hands-on ABCDEs

Perform the hands-on ABCDEs (Appearance, Breathing, Circulation, Disability, and Everything else) to determine if the ambulance service should be called and what first aid care is needed.

(5) First Aid Care

Provide first aid care appropriate to the injury or illness.

(6) Notify

As soon as possible, notify the child's parent(s) or legal guardian(s).

(7) Debrief

As soon as possible, talk with the child who received first aid about any concerns he or she may have, and talk with other children who witnessed the injury and first aid procedures.

(8) Document

Complete an incident report form.

(9) Prevention

Immediately remove or fence off any obvious danger. If this is not possible, report the hazard appropriately and place suitable signage up as an interim measure.

What You Should Do

First Aid Care for Convulsive Seizures

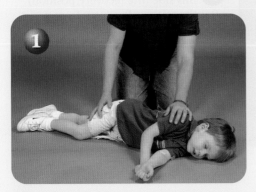

1 Position the child on his side to allow saliva to drain, and to keep the tongue from blocking the airway. Positioning the child on his left side reduces the risk of blocking the airway if vomiting occurs.

2 Loosen any restrictive clothing. Perform rescue breathing if the child is blue or is not breathing.

3 Never put anything into the child's mouth.

4 Move toys and furniture out of the way. Identify another adult to supervise the other children and explain to them that you are helping the child.

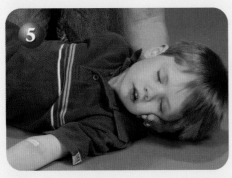

5 Slide the palm of your hand under the child's head to protect the head from injury if possible. You can also protect the child's head with a towel, blanket, or clothing. Do not try to hold the head still as this may cause further injury.

6 Note the time the seizure begins and ends and observe the body parts affected. A seizure might seem to last longer than it actually does, especially if you are frightened. Your detailed description of what happened just before, during, and after the seizure is important information to give to the child's general practitioner.

7 Call the ambulance service if the child has no seizure history and you do not have other instructions for what to do when this child has a seizure. Always notify the parent(s) or legal guardian(s) when a seizure occurs, even if the child is known to have seizures.

First Aid Care for Convulsive Seizures (cont.)

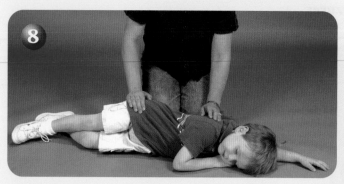

8 Let the child rest, while lying on his side (the recovery position) after the seizure. Recovery from a seizure is usually slow. The child will sleep or be drowsy for a while. Occasionally, children will be overactive following a seizure.

9 A child who is known to have seizures should have a care plan for seizures. Follow this plan and call the child's parent(s) or legal guardian(s).

What You Should Do

First Aid Care for Non-Convulsive Seizures

1 Time the seizure and observe the body parts affected if movements occur.

2 Make sure the child is in a place where he will not be injured if he moves during the seizure.

3 Let the child rest if needed.

4 A child who is known to have seizures should have a care plan. Follow this plan and call the child's parent(s) or legal guardian(s).

First Aid Tip

- Do not force anything between the child's teeth.
- Do not restrain the child's movements.
- Protect the child from his environment.
- Do not give anything to eat or drink until the child is fully alert.

Algorithm

First Aid for Seizures

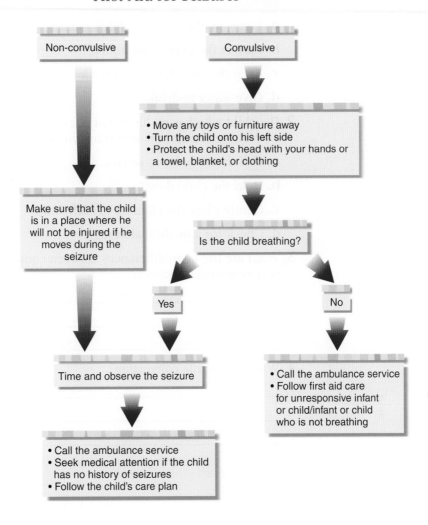

Non-convulsive

Convulsive

- Move any toys or furniture away
- Turn the child onto his left side
- Protect the child's head with your hands or a towel, blanket, or clothing

Make sure that the child is in a place where he will not be injured if he moves during the seizure

Is the child breathing?

Yes

No

Time and observe the seizure

- Call the ambulance service
- Follow first aid care for unresponsive infant or child/infant or child who is not breathing

- Call the ambulance service
- Seek medical attention if the child has no history of seizures
- Follow the child's care plan

Check Your Knowledge

1. When caring for a child who is experiencing a seizure, you should:

   a. Force an object in the child's mouth.

   b. Protect the child from injury.

   c. Keep the child flat on her back.

   d. Give water to drink.

2. If a child who has no history of seizures begins to have a convulsive seizure, the first thing you should do is:

   a. Call the ambulance service.

   b. Hold the child down.

   c. Gently place the child on her left side.

   d. Check for a medical alert tag.

3. What are the main differences between convulsive and non-convulsive seizures?

   _____

   _____

   _____

4. What is a febrile convulsion?

   _____

   _____

   _____

Terms

Aura	A feeling that indicates that a seizure is about to begin.
Convulsive seizures	Seizures characterised by involuntary muscle contractions and body movement.
Febrile convulsion	Convulsive seizure that is caused by a rapid rise in body temperature.
Non-convulsive seizures	Seizures that are associated with confusion and loss of awareness.
Partial seizures	Non-convulsive seizures that are characterised by a brief loss of consciousness.
Seizures	Disturbances in the electrical impulses of the brain that result in a variety of body responses.
Tonic-clonic seizure	Convulsive seizure that involves the entire body.

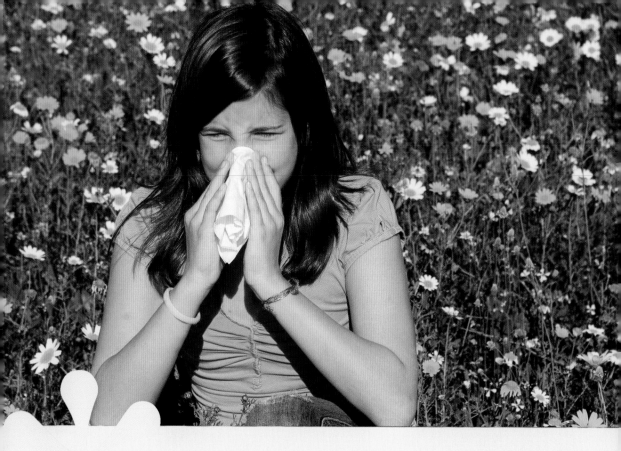

Learning Objectives

The participant will be able to:

- Recognise a child who is having an allergic reaction.
- Identify anaphylactic shock.
- Identify appropriate first aid for a child who is having an allergic reaction.
- Identify appropriate first aid for a child who is experiencing anaphylactic shock.
- Describe the skills required for using an auto-injector (containing adrenaline) for a child who has been prescribed an auto-injector (containing adrenaline) for allergic emergencies.

Chapter

8

Allergic Reactions

Allergic Reactions

Introduction

An **allergy** is the body's negative reaction to an allergen. An **allergen** is a substance that the body perceives as dangerous. Some common allergens are moulds, dust, animal dander, pollen, foods, medications, cleaning products, and other chemicals. Allergens trigger **allergic reactions**. These reactions are usually characterised by hives or tissue swelling (**Figure 8-1**). Some of the more common symptoms are runny nose, watery eyes, itchy throat, coughing and wheezing, rashes, and hives. Although it is uncommon, allergies can cause **anaphylaxis**, which causes the airway to swell and can be life-threatening.

If a child has known allergies, parent(s) or legal guardian(s) should provide written instructions on potential allergens and what to do if the child has an allergic reaction. Some children will have a prescription for antihistamine or asthma medicine to treat an allergic reaction. Carers must know how and when to use these prescribed medications. Medications should be used only for the child for whom it is prescribed and only with both a health professional's instruction and a parent's or legal guardian's consent.

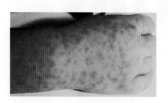

Figure 8-1

An allergic reaction can cause hives.

If a child's health professional thinks the child is at risk for anaphylactic reaction, the child's parent or legal guardian should provide an auto-injector of a medication called **adrenaline**. Adrenaline is a hormone that stops the airway from swelling. Adrenaline in an auto-injector is often marketed as Epi-Pen and Epi-Pen, Jr (**Figure 8-2**). The auto-injector must be prescribed by a health professional. Carers who are expected to use an auto-injector must receive training from a health professional.

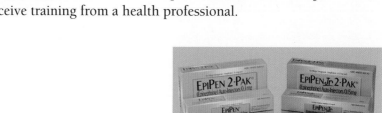

Figure 8-2

Epi-Pen.

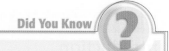

Did You Know

Allergic symptoms may include itchy eyes, runny nose, cough, rash, trouble breathing, vomiting, or diarrhoea. The child's health professional may write a prescription for an antihistamine and list the symptoms that indicate when to give this medication. A parent or legal guardian must also sign a permission form. A single dose of prescribed antihistamine upon a phone approval from the child's parent or legal guardian can stop an allergic reaction before it becomes severe.

What You Should Know

Anaphylaxis is a severe allergic reaction and a type of shock that can be fatal if not reversed within minutes. Anaphylaxis occurs suddenly, usually within seconds or minutes after a child comes in contact with the allergen. Anaphylaxis can cause airway swelling that cuts off the child's ability to breathe. If adrenaline is not available, death can occur within minutes.

Anaphylaxis can be unexpected because the child or carer may be unaware of the child's extreme allergy to a substance that is harmless to most people. Anaphylaxis is a rare type of allergic reaction. It is more likely to be caused by insect stings or food allergies than by environmental allergens such as moulds, dust, animal dander, and pollen.

Anaphylaxis more often occurs in a child who has been exposed at least once, and usually multiple times to one of the following substances:

- Insect stings from bees, wasps, or hornets
- A medication
- A food, such as shellfish, nuts, eggs, or milk

Usually, anaphylaxis is not the first type of allergic reaction a child will experience when exposed to one of these substances. However, the exposures that trigger an allergic reaction might not be obvious. A child might eat a prepared food without knowing that it contains an allergic ingredient.

Did You Know

Shock is a condition that can be caused by numerous factors (dehydration, allergic reactions, loss of blood, infection). The general treatment for shock is to call the ambulance service and keep the child warm and calm. The child should lie down with their feet slightly elevated, unless you suspect a spinal injury. The child who may be experiencing shock should also be covered with a blanket to maintain warmth and attempt to control any further loss of blood. If the child has an adrenaline auto-injector, it may also be helpful to assist in administering this medication if the shock is related to an allergy.

Did You Know

Common food allergies:
- Chocolate
- Eggs
- Milk
- Nuts
- Peanuts
- Shellfish
- Soya beans
- Wheat

Did You Know

An allergy can develop at any time in life, no matter how often a person was previously exposed to the substance.

Children who have had an extreme allergic reaction to a specific allergen should have an auto-injector containing adrenaline. Store the auto-injector device at room temperature with the first aid supplies. An auto-injector is not a routine item in first aid kits; it is a prescription drug intended only for the child with allergies in an emergency. The auto-injector is an easy-to-use device that administers the correct dose of adrenaline. The auto-injector must always be close at hand wherever the child goes. If the child goes farther away from the storage place for the auto-injector than nearby rooms in the child care facility, the auto-injector should go with the child. This means carers should carry the device out to the playground with the first aid supplies and on field trips.

Did You Know

All ambulances should carry adrenaline auto-injectors, however do not wait for the ambulance to arrive if the child is having a severe anaphylactic reaction. Given as per the instructions, the benefits of this life-saving drug completely outweigh any risks.

Children allergic to certain foods can usually be protected from exposure. Sharing of food must not be allowed. Some child care settings restrict foods that children can bring into the facility and attempt to educate all parents and legal guardians about how to avoid foods that have ingredients harmful to a classmate with allergies. There is some danger in this, however, because it is difficult to educate all of the carers who may prepare foods for a child.

Separating a child with allergies from her classmates during snack and meal times may be appropriate in severe cases, but it can make the child feel isolated. Arrange for a member of the staff to supervise a small group that includes one or two friends and the child who has a food allergy when she must be separated from the rest of the children who are eating foods that might pose a hazard. Be aware that some children with allergies are so sensitive that even touching a surface that has been touched by someone eating a food that contains the allergen can trigger an allergic response. The only way to protect such children is to ban the food from the environment of that child altogether.

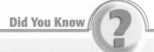

Did You Know

Visit www.allergyinschools.org.uk for a wide range of information and resources for parents, carers, and teachers for pre-school or older school-age groups.

What You Should Look For

Symptoms include:

- Swelling of the face, lips, and throat
- Wheezing/shortness of breath
- Tightness in the chest
- Dizziness
- Blue/grey colour around lips
- Nausea and vomiting
- Drooling
- Itchy skin, hives, or other rashes appearing quickly

What You Should Do

The Nine Steps in Paediatric First Aid:

1 Survey the Scene

Take a brief moment to perform a scene survey to ensure that the scene is safe, to find out who is involved, and to determine what happened.

2 Hands-off ABCs

As you approach the child, perform the hands-off ABCs (Appearance, Breathing, and Circulation) to determine if the ambulance service should be called. It should take 15 to 30 seconds or less.

3 Supervise

Immediately ensure that any other children near the scene are properly supervised.

4 Hands-on ABCDEs

Perform the hands-on ABCDEs (Appearance, Breathing, Circulation, Disability, and Everything else) to determine if the ambulance service should be called and what first aid care is needed.

5 First Aid Care

Provide first aid care appropriate to the injury or illness.

6 Notify

As soon as possible, notify the child's parent(s) or legal guardian(s).

7 Debrief

As soon as possible, talk with the child who received first aid about any concerns he or she may have, and talk with other children who witnessed the injury and first aid procedures.

8 Document

Complete an incident report form.

9 Prevention

Immediately remove or fence off any obvious danger. If this is not possible, report the hazard appropriately and place suitable signage up as an interim measure.

What You Should Do

First Aid Care for Anaphylaxis

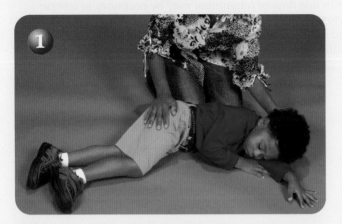

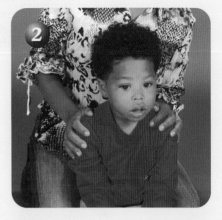

1 Place an unresponsive child on his left side. Check for breathing and call the ambulance service. If the child is not breathing, follow the steps outlined on page 36.

2 Place a conscious child who is having trouble breathing in a sitting position to make breathing easier, and call the ambulance service.

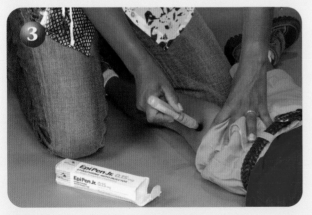
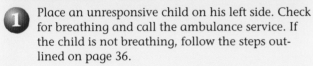

3 If a child has an adrenaline auto-injector, administer it immediately as intended by the manufacturer and according to the instructions of the child's health care professional. A second injection may be needed if the ambulance service does not arrive within 5 minutes of the first injection. If the child does not have an auto-injector, monitor ABCs and treat symptoms accordingly. Administer asthma medication or antihistamine if it is prescribed by the child's health care professional and you have parental consent. Parent(s) or legal guardian(s) should be notified of any allergic reaction.

Did You Know ?

- More than one dose of adrenaline may be necessary to reverse anaphylaxis.
- A second dose can be given after 5 minutes if necessary.
- Adrenaline can cause a rapid heart rate, pale skin, and nausea.

Algorithm

First Aid Care for Allergy or Anaphylaxis

Seek immediate medical attention. Activate the ambulance service if reaction is severe or if auto-injector will be used

Does the child have an auto-injector available?

No

Yes

Monitor ABCs and treat accordingly

Administer adrenaline auto-injector according to kit's directions

Administer asthma medication or antihistamine if child is conscious and child's health professional has prescribed the medication with parent/legal guardian consent

Continue checking child while waiting for the ambulance service to arrive. A second injection may be needed if the ambulance service does not arrive within 5 minutes of the first injection

Check Your Knowledge

1. A child has been stung by a bee. Within minutes her face and tongue are swelling and she is having difficulty breathing. These signs and symptoms are associated with:

   a. Seizures

   b. Anaphylaxis

   c. Asthma

   d. Hypoglycaemia

2. Sharing of food with a child who has food allergies:

   a. Is acceptable if the food is baked

   b. Is a healthy way for children to learn to share

   c. Must not be allowed

   d. Is acceptable on holidays

3. List the main signs and symptoms for a child suffering from an anaphylactic reaction.

   _____

   _____

   _____

4. What is an anaphylactic reaction?

   _____

   _____

   _____

Terms

Adrenaline	A hormone that stops the effects of anaphylaxis.
Allergen	A substance that the body perceives as dangerous.
Allergic reactions	Local or general reactions to an allergen usually characterised by hives or tissue swelling.
Allergy	A hypersensitivity to a substance, causing an abnormal reaction.
Anaphylaxis	A severe allergic reaction and a type of shock that can be fatal if not reversed within minutes.

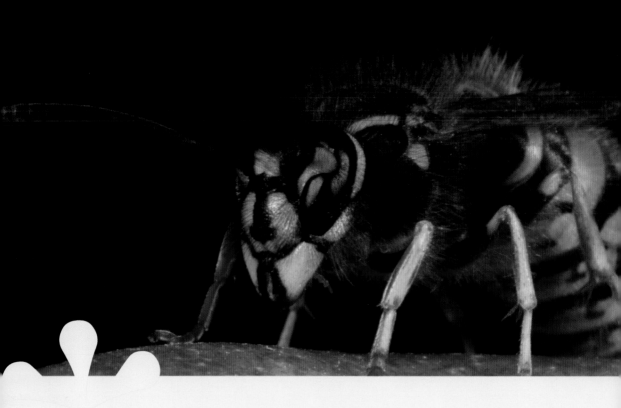

Learning Objectives

The participant will be able to:

- Recognise bites and stings.
- Identify the major risks from human and animal bites.
- Describe first aid for bites and stings.

Chapter

9

Bites and Stings

Bites and Stings

Introduction

Animal and human bites are common sources of injury to young children. Many animals and insects that can cause injury are specific to certain geographic locations. For instance, ticks are common in moor and heathland areas. You should know how to provide first aid care for common types of bites or stings in your area.

In general, most bites are more of a nuisance than a serious health problem. However, some bites can be associated with potentially serious diseases. The person giving paediatric first aid should handle bites and stings by providing the care that keeps the situation from getting worse. In some situations, a medical professional needs to evaluate and manage the injured child.

Animal and Human Bites

What You Should Know

Each year in the United Kingdom, approximately 200,000 people are bitten by dogs, with many of the bites occurring to children (**Figure 9-1**). Children under the age of 5 are susceptible to the most serious of injuries. Seventy per cent of bites are received by people's own pets. Cats are less likely to bite than dogs, but like dog bites, cat bites are likely to become infected and may cause a life-threatening situation. Exotic pets, such as ferrets and monkeys, and wild animals, such as squirrels, also bite. The teeth of an animal carry many bacteria. Any animal bite that breaks the skin can become infected and some animals may transmit disease when they bite.

The most dangerous infection that can develop after an animal bite is **rabies,** which is a viral disease. Although found in parts of Europe, the last human death from rabies was in 1922. Care should be taken when holidaying or on school trips abroad. The rabies virus is present in the saliva of an infected animal and is transmitted to a person through a bite or cross contamination with the saliva of the rabid host. This disease affects the brain and the nervous system. Once rabies symptoms develop, the disease is fatal. To ensure that this deadly illness does not develop, a medical professional must evaluate a person who has been bitten or scratched by a wild animal or by a pet that has not received a rabies vaccine. Whenever possible, try to confirm the pet's rabies vaccine status from the pet's owner. Never try to capture or restrain the pet in question.

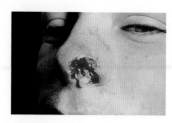

Figure 9-1

Dog bite.

Human bites are common in groups of toddlers. Biting is a non-verbal child's way of expressing anger or frustration. Many of these bites are minor and do not break the skin. They cause more of an emotional upset than a physical injury. As with an animal bite, when a human bite breaks the skin, the risk of infection is significant.

What You Should Look For

- Superficial skin breaks with little or no bleeding
- Puncture-type wounds
- Lacerations
- Crushing injuries
- Torn tissues in the area of the bite

What You Should Do

The Nine Steps in Paediatric First Aid:

1 Survey the Scene

Take a brief moment to perform a scene survey to ensure that the scene is safe, to find out who is involved, and to determine what happened.

2 Hands-off ABCs

As you approach the child, perform the hands-off ABCs (<u>A</u>ppearance, <u>B</u>reathing, and <u>C</u>irculation) to determine if the ambulance service should be called. It should take 15 to 30 seconds or less.

3 Supervise

Immediately ensure that any other children near the scene are properly supervised.

4 Hands-on ABCDEs

Perform the hands-on ABCDEs (<u>A</u>ppearance, <u>B</u>reathing, <u>C</u>irculation, <u>D</u>isability, and <u>E</u>verything else) to determine if the ambulance service should be called and what first aid care is needed.

5 First Aid Care

Provide first aid care appropriate to the injury or illness.

6 Notify

As soon as possible, notify the child's parent(s) or legal guardian(s).

7 Debrief

As soon as possible, talk with the child who received first aid about any concerns he or she may have, and talk with other children who witnessed the injury and first aid procedures.

8 Document

Complete an incident report form.

9 Prevention

Immediately remove or fence off any obvious danger. If this is not possible, report the hazard appropriately and place suitable signage up as an interim measure.

What You Should Do

First Aid Care for Bites from Dogs, Cats, Other Animals, and Humans

 Remove the child and others from area. If the bite caused serious injury or uncontrollable bleeding, call the ambulance service immediately. If the injury was caused by an animal bite whilst abroad, seek urgent medical attention.

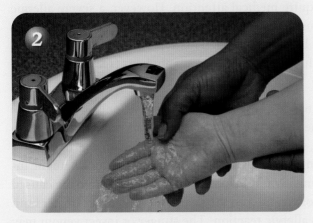

 Care for any wound or bruised area. Be sure to thoroughly wash with soap and rinse with water any areas where the skin was scratched, punctured, or cut to reduce the risk of infection. If the skin is not broken, clean the area with soap and water, apply a cold pack over a cloth to protect the skin, and comfort the child who was bitten.

 Although not a bite, scratches from animals such as domestic cats can posses a high risk of infection. Any such scratch should be assessed by a health care professional as soon as possible.

Insect Bites and Stings

What You Should Know

Childhood encounters with bees, wasps, and hornets can be a natural consequence of children's curiosity and exploration (**Figure 9-2A-B**). Also, children may have residue of food on their clothes or hands that attracts insects. In most cases, insect stings do not require medical attention. However, a severe allergic reaction to an insect sting can occur very quickly, without warning, and can be life-threatening. This type of severe allergic reaction that is life-threatening is called anaphylaxis (see Allergic Reactions, page 114).

Venomous insects are generally aggressive only when threatened or when their hives or nests are disturbed. Under such conditions, they sting, sometimes in swarms. Children inadvertently may threaten a stinging insect by running into it or playing where the insects are swarming. Symptoms of an insect sting or bite are caused by the injection of venom into the skin. The venom can trigger both irritation and an allergic reaction. The stinger or insect venom may also cause infection.

Figure 9-2

A. Honeybee.
B. Hornet.

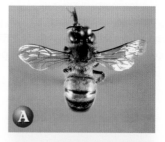

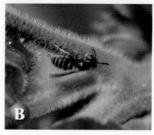

Normal reactions to an insect sting include pain, itching, and swelling that disappears in a day or so. Mild allergic reactions include hives and swelling. Although these symptoms could indicate a severe reaction for someone with anaphylaxis or asthma. Severe allergic reactions vary in intensity and usually occur within minutes to several hours after contact with the insect venom. A person who has a severe allergy to an insect sting or bite may have a prescribed auto-injector of adrenaline.

Biting insects include mosquitoes, gnats, midges, and some types of flies. In many areas of the country, these insects can transmit diseases that are specific to that area. The insects inject the germs that cause the infection along with their saliva when they puncture the skin. Usually, these insect bites itch and are annoying for a few days, but cause no other problems.

First Aid Tip

**Using an Auto-Injector of Adrenaline
for Severe Allergic Reactions**
- Call the ambulance service
- Do not remove the safety cap until you are ready to use the medication.
- Never put your fingers over the black ejection tip while removing the grey safety cap or after you have administered the medication.
- Do not use the auto-injector if :
  - It is not prescribed to the patient
  - It is discoloured (yellow versus clear)
  - Has particles in it
  - It is past the expiration date printed on the side of the box
- Hold the auto-injector in your hand and make a fist around it. Remove the auto-injector's safety cap.
- Place the black tip of the injector directly against the patient's outer thigh (you can inject through clothing). Do not inject the medication into the vein or the buttocks. Inject it into the fleshy outer portion of the thigh.
- With a rapid motion, push the auto-injector firmly against the thigh and hold it in place until all the medication is injected— usually no more than 10 seconds.
- Remove the injector and replace it into its safety tube, and give it to the ambulance personnel upon their arrival.
- Massage the injection area after it has been properly administered.

Mosquitoes and gnats are most active around dawn and dusk, as well as when it is humid. Midges are small winged biting insects found throughout the whole United Kingdom, but are infamous in parts of Scotland. They are attracted to dark-coloured clothing and are prominent at dusk and dawn. Their bites are more irritating than dangerous.

Although some insects can bite, most avoid contact with people. Some insects are attractive to children, even though they would rather be left alone. For example, children love to handle caterpillars although many caterpillars can cause a rash.

What You Should Look For

- Painful or itchy area where the insect stung or bit the child
- Redness and swelling in the area of the sting or bite
- Child feeling or acting ill
- Signs of an allergic reaction, such as:
  - Hives, extensive swelling, or spreading rash
  - Difficulty breathing
  - A dry, hacking cough, wheezing, or tightness in nose, throat, or chest
  - Itchy eyes
  - Swelling of lips, eyes, or throat
  - Weakness or dizziness
  - Rapid heartbeat
  - Nausea/vomiting

What You Should Do

First Aid Care for Mild to Moderate Reactions to Insect Stings and Bites

1 Move the child to a safe area to avoid more stings or bites.

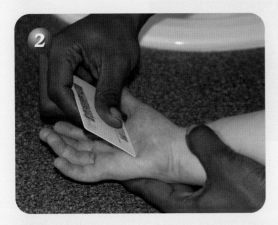

2 Remove any body parts of the stinging or biting insect. Look for and quickly remove any stinger by scraping it with a credit card or fingernail. If the child has touched a caterpillar that left any of its spines on the skin, remove the spines with the sticky side of tape.

3 Wash the area with soap and rinse with water.

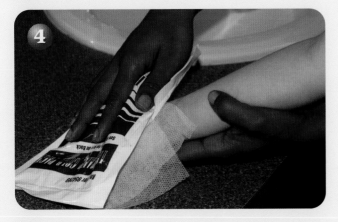

4 Apply a cold pack over a cloth to protect the skin to reduce pain and swelling.

First Aid Care for Mild to Moderate Reactions to Insect Stings and Bites (cont.)

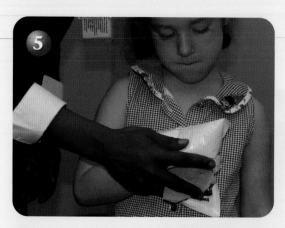

5 Keep the area elevated (above the heart).

6 If the child has an antihistamine or other medication that has been prescribed for insect bites or stings and the parent(s) or legal guardian(s) has given written consent for using it, give the medication right away. If you administered a prescribed auto-injector, contact the ambulance service immediately. (See Allergic Reactions, page 114.)

7 Observe the child for any additional reaction to the bite or sting, and to the medication.

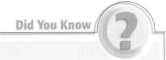

Honeybees leave a sack attached to their stinger in the skin. The sack continues to pump venom into the bite site for a few seconds after the sting. Getting it out right away can reduce the amount of venom that irritates the tissues. Hornets and some wasps also leave a stinger in the skin. Since stingers can carry many bacteria, taking stingers out reduces the risk of infection.

Avoiding Insect Stings

- Check for nests in locations where children play, such as in old tree stumps, in car tyres that are part of a playground, in holes in the ground, around rubbish bins, and around rotting wood.
- Have insect nests removed by professional exterminators.
- Children who are allergic to insects should not play outside alone when stinging insects are active.
- Wear shoes and avoid wearing sandals or going barefoot.
- Avoid wearing bright colours and floral patterns on clothing because these can attract insects. White, green, tan, and khaki are the least attractive colours to insects.
- When eating outdoors, avoid foods that attract insects such as: tuna, peanut butter and jam sandwiches, watermelon, sweetened drinks, lollipops, and ice cream.
- Avoid being near rubbish bins and dumpsters.
- If an insect is near, do not swat at it or run. These actions can trigger an attack. Walk away slowly. If you have disturbed a nest and the insects swarm around you, curl up as tightly as you can to reduce exposed skin, keep your face down and cover your head with your arms.
- A child who is allergic to insects should wear a medical alert necklace or bracelet.

Tick Bites

What You Should Know

A tick is a tiny brown mite that attaches itself to the skin of an animal or human and sucks blood (**Figures 9-3** and **9-4 A-B**). Ticks do not fly or jump; they attach themselves to an animal or human who brushes up against them. Diseases carried by ticks include Lyme disease which has severly debilitating side effects; however, most tick bites do not cause disease.

Ticks must feed on blood to survive. It is during these feedings that disease can be transmitted to humans. As the tick feeds, it deposits the waste from its gut in the wound where it is feeding. Infection is less likely to occur if the tick is removed before it has time to feed and fill with blood. The risk of being bitten by an infected tick is greatest in the summer months, especially in May and June, but in some areas ticks can be a year-round threat. Warm weather months are the time of year when children are most active outdoors.

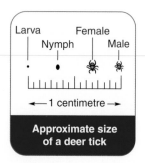

Figure 9-3

Scale of a deer tick.

What You Should Look For

- An embedded tick or a bump on the skin that is new

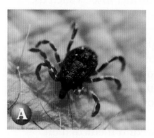
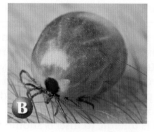

Figure 9-4

A. A deer tick that is not engorged (filled with blood).
B. One that is engorged.

What You Should Do

First Aid Care for Tick Bites

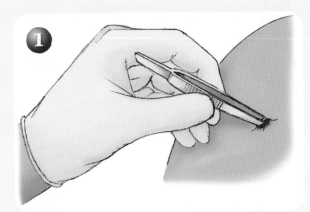

1 Pull an embedded tick out using tweezers.

2 Grasp the tick as close to the skin as possible and lift it in the direction in which the tick appears to have entered, pulling with enough force to "tent" the skin surface. Hold it in that position until the tick lets go. This may take several seconds. Do not twist or jerk the tick, which may result in incomplete removal. Do not grab a tick at the rear of its body. The body of the tick may rupture and the infectious contents may be squeezed into the wound made by the tick's bite.

3 Wash the bite area with warm soap and water.

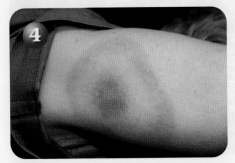

4 For several weeks, watch the bitten area for a rash. If a rash appears, or the child becomes ill, the child's parent(s) or legal guardian(s) should take the child to a medical professional.

5 Inform the parent(s) or legal guardian(s) that you have removed a tick from the child so they are able to watch the child for any reaction that may occur.

First Aid Tip

Do not use any of the following ineffective methods of tick removal:

- Petroleum jelly
- Fingernail polish
- Surgical spirit
- Kerosene or petrol
- A match head that is blown out but is still hot

Snakebites

What You Should Know

Snakebites are quite rare in the United Kingdom (UK) and non-existent in Ireland. The majority of incidents involve the adder, which is the UK's only native venomous snake (**Figure 9-5**). Adder bites usually occur in the summer months, and usually to

Figure 9-5

Adder.

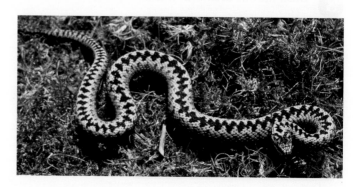

people who are walking through areas of long grass, sand dunes, or heathland. Smooth snakes and grass snakes are very common, but non-venomous.

What You Should Look For

- Two small puncture wounds a couple of centimetres apart (some cases may have only one fang mark)
- Child complaining of severe burning pain at the bite site
- Rapid swelling
- Discolouration and blood-filled blisters (may develop within 6 to 10 hours)
- In severe cases, nausea, vomiting, sweating, and generalised weakness

What You Should Do

First Aid Care for Snakebites

1 Get child and others away from the snake.

2 Keep the child quiet and the body part still to slow the spread of venom. The bitten arm or leg should be kept at or lower than the child's heart to keep the venom from spreading in the body.

3 It is often helpful to immobilise the limb, similar to when treating a fractured limb. This helps to keep the area still. Call the ambulance service.

First Aid Tip

- Do not use mouth suction because the human mouth is filled with bacteria, which increases the chance of wound infection.
- Do not apply a constricting band around an arm or leg since it can cause additional injury.
- Call the ambulance service immediately.

Spider Bites

What You Should Know

In the UK and Ireland, spiders are not normally considered hazardous to health. It is now recognized that around a dozen native species exist that are capable of inflicting a significant bite. However, the reports of annual bites are only just into double figures and just as many cases relate to bites from exotic pets. A spider bite is often difficult to recognize, especially when the spider was not seen or recovered, because the bites typically cause little immediate pain.

What You Should Look For

- Tiny fang marks
- Pain begins as a dull ache at the bite site
- Blister at the bite site
- Mild swelling and lightening of skin colour at the site of the bite
- Progressive soft tissue damage

What You Should Do

First Aid Care for Spider Bites

 If a child is bitten by a spider, wash the bite with soap and water.

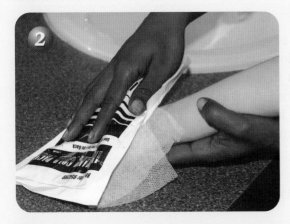

 Apply an ice pack over a cloth on the bite site to relieve pain and delay the effects of the venom.

 Take the child to an accident and emergency department, minor injuries unit, or call the ambulance service.

Marine Animal Stings

What You Should Know

Most marine animals bite or sting in defence. Jellyfish are responsible for more stings than any other marine animal in the seas around Britain.

The weever fish is very hard to see, but as many seaside-goers find out each year at low tide, they are easy to step on (**Figure 9-6**). The fish buries itself in sandy areas where the water is warm and shallow. It has five to seven spines that protrude from its back. These poisonous spines are left exposed above the surface of the sand and have even been known to penetrate wetsuit boots.

What You Should Look For

- Swelling
- Small pin-prick holes

Figure 9-6

Weever fish.

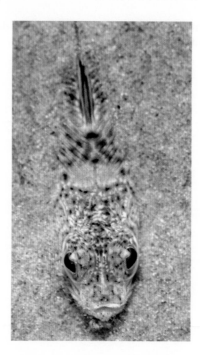

What You Should Do

First Aid Care for Marine Animal Stings

1 Remove the child from the water.

2 Rinse the skin with sea water.

3 If the injury is caused by a sting, pour vinegar on the affected area until pain is relieved. Unlike fresh water, vinegar will render the nematocysts inactive.

4 Attempt to remove the loose tentacles by scraping them off with the edge of a sharp, stiff object such as a credit card or forceps. Do not handle tentacles with bare hands.

5 If the injury is caused by weever spines, immerse the injured part in hot water (as hot as can be tolerated) for 30 to 90 minutes.

6 Wash the wound with soap and water, and then flush the area with water under pressure to wash out as much of the toxin and foreign material as possible.

7 Seek medical advice for pain and swelling.

Algorithm

First Aid Care for Animal Bites

First, remove child and others from area

If the bite has caused serious injury or uncontrollable bleeding, call the ambulance service

Care for any wound or bruise, washing and rinsing any opening in the skin thoroughly

For any bite or scratch, seek clinical assessment as soon as possible

---

First Aid Care for Insect Bites and Stings, and Tick Bites

Move the child and any others away from the location where the insects are active

Remove any stinger or body parts of the insect or tick that are attached. Use a credit card or fingernail to scrape out stingers; use tweezers at the attachment of a tick to the skin; use sticky tape to pick up caterpillar spines

Wash any opening in the skin with soap/and rinse with running water

Apply cold and elevate to control pain and swelling in the area of the bite or sting

Give any prescribed medication for children who are known to have allergic reactions

First Aid Care for Snake and Spider Bites

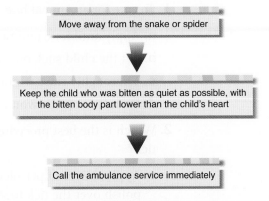

Move away from the snake or spider

Keep the child who was bitten as quiet as possible, with the bitten body part lower than the child's heart

Call the ambulance service immediately

First Aid Care for Marine Animal Bites

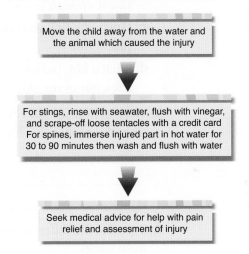

Move the child away from the water and the animal which caused the injury

For stings, rinse with seawater, flush with vinegar, and scrape-off loose tentacles with a credit card
For spines, immerse injured part in hot water for 30 to 90 minutes then wash and flush with water

Seek medical advice for help with pain relief and assessment of injury

Check Your Knowledge

1. To care for an animal bite:

a. Apply antibiotic ointment over the bite area.

b. Let the child suck on small bite wounds.

c. Thoroughly rinse wound with soap and water.

d. Do not cover the wound so air can dry the wound.

2. Which is the best procedure for removing an embedded tick?

a. Apply a layer of petroleum jelly, peanut butter or nail polish over the tick to smother it

b. Apply several drops of surgical spirit on the tick to irritate it enough to back out

c. Grasp the tick with tweezers close to the skin and gently pull it out

d. Stick a hot, blown-out match to the tick to cause it to back out of the skin

3. What action should you take for a child who has been stung by a jellyfish while on a school trip?

_____

_____

_____

4. Describe the different procedures for dealing with bee and wasp stings.

_____

_____

_____

Terms

Rabies   A life-threatening viral disease in warm-blooded mammals that is primarily transferred through bites, now eradicated in the UK.

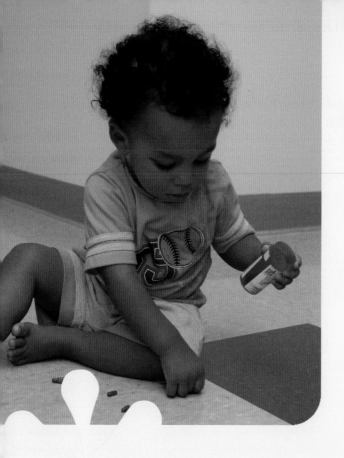

Learning Objectives

The participant will be able to:

- Recognise a child who has swallowed, contacted, or inhaled poison.
- Identify appropriate first aid for a child who has swallowed poison.
- Identify appropriate first aid for a child who has inhaled poison.
- Identify appropriate first aid for a child who has had contact with a poisonous plant(s).

Chapter

10 Poisoning

Poisoning

Introduction

A **poison** is a substance that, when swallowed, inhaled, or absorbed through the skin can cause damage to the body, illness, and sometimes death. Often exposure to only a tiny amount of a poisonous substance can have serious consequences. Poisoning is one of the most common causes of injury in children under 5 years of age.

What You Should Know

Many products that are used daily are highly toxic and potentially fatal. They can have tragic consequences when swallowed. In general, the poisonous substances that are most devastating to children are medications, cleaning products, pesticides, alcoholic beverages, and petroleum products.

Young children are curious by nature. Coloured plastic containers, colourful pills, and never-before-seen-items invite the child to explore. Taste is the first sense toddlers and many preschoolers use when investigating something new, regardless of whether it is a toy, food, chemical, or plant. Poisonings often happen when adults are tired or preoccupied, when children have been left alone (even momentarily), and when proper storage or disposal of a poison is either interrupted or forgotten. Most childhood poisonings can be prevented by safe use and proper storage of household products and medicines. Keep household products and medicines in locked cabinets on high, secure shelves or in boxes that are inaccessible to children.

Like many adults, most young children know little about toxic plants. Because children use their senses of touch and taste when investigating something new, it is not unusual for them to touch and mouth leaves, berries, and flowers. Poisonings can occur from swallowing a plant, absorbing a toxin through the skin, or inhaling fumes from a fire that contains a poisonous plant. For the children's safety, learn the names of the plants, trees, and shrubbery around your facility. If a child swallows any part of a plant that you know to be poisonous or are unfamiliar with, take the child to the nearest accident and emergency (A&E) department, minor injuries unit, or call the ambulance service. Remember to take a sample of the plant with you, but be particularly cautious in handling any plant part and use a plastic bag for extra safety.

A small number of plants can cause a chemical and sometimes, an allergic reaction, when they make contact with the skin. The best known is poison ivy which is found in the United Kingdom (**Figure 10-1**).

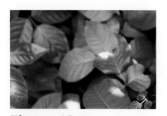

Figure 10-1

Poison ivy.

Exposure to the oil of these plants causes a chemical reaction of irritation and can cause a delayed allergic reaction in the form of a rash that varies in severity (**Figure 10-2**). A child can be exposed to the oil of the plants directly by touching the leaves, stems, or roots, or indirectly by touching tools, clothes, pets, or any other articles touched by the plant. Smoke from a fire containing the burning plant can carry this oil in tiny droplets to the skin and into the nose, throat, and lungs. A reaction can develop from contact with these plants during any season of the year and from handling any part of the plant, not just the leaves.

Poisoning by inhalation can occur as in carbon monoxide poisoning from a faulty furnace, a paraffin space heater, or a car motor running in an enclosed garage. Carbon monoxide poisoning causes rapid unconsciousness, sometimes preceded by a severe headache. It is often fatal. Inhaled poisoning also can occur if a child experiments with intentionally inhaling a chemical, such as the fumes from rubber cement or model glue.

Figure 10-2

Rash from a plant.

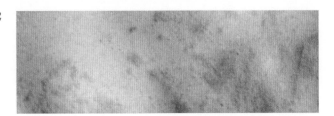

Did You Know ?

Child-resistant safety packaging for medication was developed in the 1970s. There is no such thing as "childproof packaging". However, this type of packaging does slow the child's access to the medication so that an adult has a better chance of finding the child first.

Did You Know ?

One of the leading causes of childhood poisoning is paracetamol. It is a significant cause of liver damage and even death.

What You Should Look For

Swallowed Poison:

- Opened container of medicine or chemical
- Unusual odour from mouth or clothes
- Burns in and around the mouth indicating contact with a corrosive chemical
- Nausea or vomiting
- Abdominal pain or diarrhoea
- Drowsiness
- Unconsciousness

Poisonous Plant Exposure:

- Rash
- Itching
- Redness
- Blisters
- Swelling

Inhaled Poisons:

- A source of fumes that may or may not have an odour
- Change in behaviour
- Change in appearance

What You Should Do

The Nine Steps of Paediatric First Aid:

1 Survey the Scene

Take a brief moment to perform a scene survey to ensure that the scene is safe, to find out who is involved, and to determine what happened.

2 Hands-off ABCs

As you approach the child, perform the hands-off ABCs (Appearance, Breathing, and Circulation) to determine if the ambulance service should be called. It should take 15 to 30 seconds or less.

3 Supervise

Immediately ensure that any other children near the scene are properly supervised.

4 Hands-on ABCDEs

Perform the hands-on ABCDEs (Appearance, Breathing, Circulation, Disability, and Everything else) to determine if the ambulance service should be called and what first aid care is needed.

5 First Aid Care

Provide first aid care appropriate to the injury or illness.

6 Notify

As soon as possible, notify the child's parent(s) or legal guardian(s).

7 Debrief

As soon as possible, talk with the child who received first aid about any concerns he or she may have, and talk with other children who witnessed the injury and first aid procedures.

8 Document

Complete an incident report form.

9 Prevention

Immediately remove or fence off any obvious danger. If this is not possible, report the hazard appropriately and place suitable signage up as an interim measure.

What You Should Do

First Aid Care for Swallowed Poisons

 Gather information and remain calm. Try to determine the following:

- Age and weight of the child
- What was swallowed
- Amount swallowed
- When it was swallowed
- The child's condition

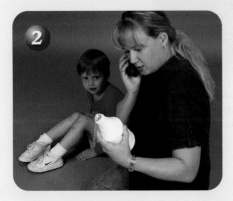

 If the child is responsive, take them to the nearest A&E department, minor injuries unit, or call the ambulance service. Take the product container with you, making sure you do not become contaminated as well. If calling the ambulance service, make sure you give details of the substance to the call taker.

First Aid Care for Swallowed Poisons (cont.)

3 If the child is unresponsive, call the ambulance service and follow the steps in Difficulty Breathing (page 36).

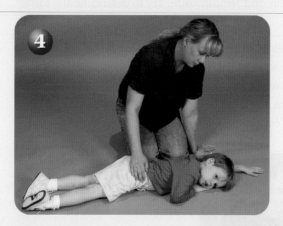

4 Place the child on his side. Lying on the left side may slow the emptying of the stomach contents. This position also keeps the airway open and allows vomit to drain from the mouth.

What You Should Do

First Aid Care for Exposure to Poisonous Plants

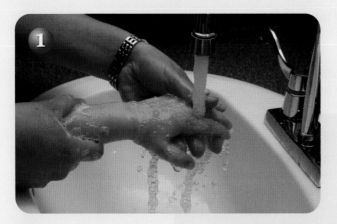

1 If a child's skin is exposed to one of these plants, immediately wash the area with soap and flush with running water to rinse off the plant oil. If a child's eye or mouth is involved, flush with water. Where possible, wear gloves yourself.

2 You may wish to call an advice line (in the United Kingdom this is provided by NHS Direct) or you can take the child and a sample of the plant to the nearest A&E department or call the ambulance service.

What You Should Do

First Aid Care for Exposure to Inhaled Poisons

1   Remove the child from a toxic area and call the ambulance service.

2   If the child is responsive, place them in a safe, comfortable position. Call the ambulance service.

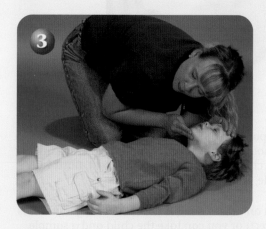

3   If the child is unresponsive, follow the steps for difficulty breathing (See Chapter 3). Be careful not to become contaminated yourself.

Algorithm

First Aid Care for a Swallowed Poison

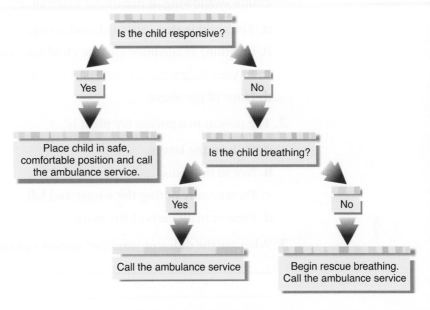

First Aid Care for an Inhaled Poison

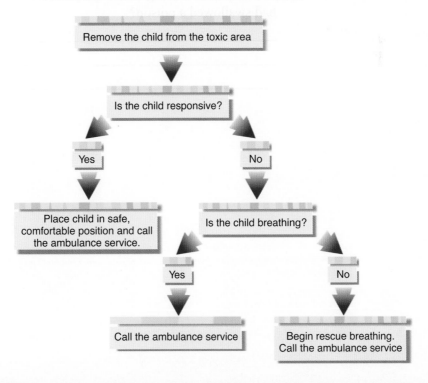

Check Your Knowledge

1. It is unnecessary to call the ambulance service following a child's swallowing of poisonous material if:

   a. The child is alert, oriented, and crying.

   b. Breathing is adequate and the child has good colour.

   c. In your judgment, a small, safe amount was swallowed.

   d. None of the above.

2. The poison in a poison ivy plant is:

   a. Only in the leaves.

   b. Not in the roots.

   c. Present only during the winter and fall.

   d. Present in all parts of the plant.

3. What are the different ways that poison can enter the body?

   _____

   _____

   _____

4. What are the main signs and symptoms for a child who had swallowed a poison?

   _____

   _____

   _____

Terms

Poison   A substance that, when swallowed, inhaled, or absorbed through the skin (from a plant), can cause illness, damage, and sometimes death.

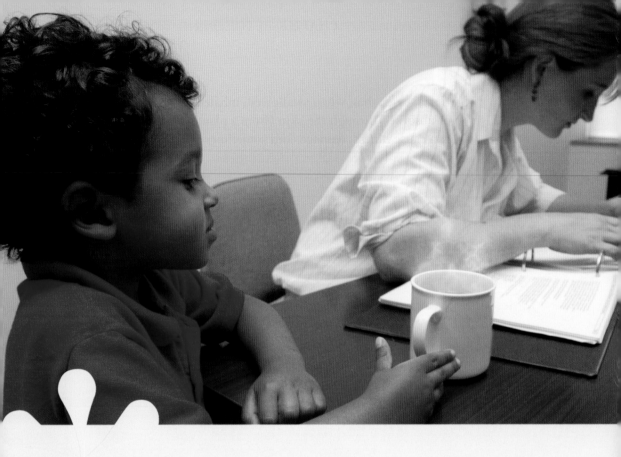

Learning Objectives

The participant will be able to:

- Identify those burns that can be addressed by first aid and those that cannot.
- Describe appropriate first aid for burns.
- Identify the symptoms of electric shock.
- Describe the appropriate first aid for electric shock.

Chapter 11

Burns

Burns

Introduction

A **burn** is an injury to the skin caused by heat, extreme cold, radiation, a chemical, or electrical damage to the body (**Figure 11-1**). Heat sources include hot water or steam, hot surfaces, and flames. Chemical burns are caused by corrosive or caustic chemicals. The most common type of radiation burn is sunburn, which is caused by ultraviolet light. Contact with electricity causes electrical burns. Burn injuries can be very painful and may take a long time to heal. A serious burn injury can leave a child with long-term physical and emotional scars.

Figure 11-1

A burn is an injury to the skin.

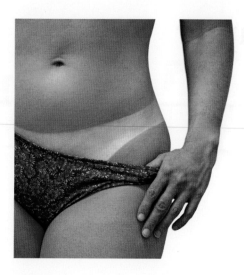

What You Should Know

Most burns to toddlers and preschoolers are scald injuries caused by hot liquids, fats, or oils. Infants are less likely to be burned than older children due to their immobility. Burns caused by flames occur more frequently to children 5 to 12 years of age. Fires that create a lot of smoke can be damaging because the chemicals in the smoke can cause severe injury to the lining of the airway and lungs.

Did You Know ?

To minimise the risk of scalding, temperature of hot water supplies to baths and showers should not exceed 43°C in many educational and care settings. Domestic water is often stored at a hotter temperature.

Corrosive or caustic chemicals cause burns by destroying the skin that comes into direct contact with the chemical. The longer the chemical is in contact with the body, the more damage it does. Some examples of corrosive or caustic chemicals are bleach, drain cleaner, and battery acids. The chemical labels will tell you whether they can cause burns. These hazardous chemicals should be stored and used carefully and should be inaccessible to children.

Children are very curious and can come upon electrical dangers, such as electrical sockets and wires from appliances, while exploring (**Figure 11-2**). Toddlers may attempt to place an object, such as a fork, in an electrical socket. Infants may chew on wires. Usually children are knocked away by the strong muscle contractions that occur after contact with electricity. However, these muscle contractions can also make the child hold on to the object instead of being knocked away, thus causing more damage.

Depending on the amount of electricity, injuries can range from a minimal reddening of the skin to severe damage to the body. An electrical burn may cause substantial deep tissue injury while showing little damage on the surface of the skin. Usually, electrical shock from a household current is not life-threatening. Nevertheless, electrical shock can cause the heart to stop. If the child who is injured by electricity is still in contact with the source of the electrical current, the electricity can flow to and injure any person who touches the child.

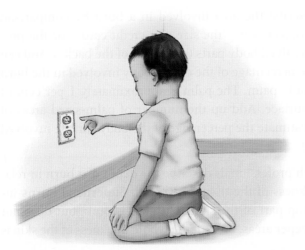

Figure 11-2

Electrical outlets should have protective devices to prevent injury.

People who have a history of one or more blistering sunburns during childhood or adolescence are two times more likely to develop skin cancer. Chronic exposure to sunlight (ultraviolet light, UV) is the cause of most cases of skin cancer. More than half of a person's lifetime UV exposure occurs during childhood and adolescence. Protection from UV exposure reduces the risk for skin cancer. When children play outside, they should always wear sun-protective clothing, seek shade, and use sunscreen or sunblock. Sunscreen contains a chemical that bonds to the skin to prevent injury from UV light. Sunblock is a barrier cream that prevents the UV light from reaching the skin. Unlike burns from direct contact with hot surfaces, the irritation of the skin from sunburn takes time to develop.

The severity of a burn is determined by three major factors: size, location, and depth. The size, location, and depth of a burn determine whether a medical professional should be involved in care. Larger and deeper burns are more serious injuries. Burns of the face, hands, feet, or genitals are more serious than burns in other locations of the body. Unfortunately, children commonly burn their face, hands, feet, or genitals when they reach up to stovetops, touch hot appliances, or spill hot liquids in their laps. A burn that may be considered a minor injury to an adult could be a serious injury for a young child.

You can describe the area involved in a burn by comparison with a familiar object (e.g., "the size of a credit card") or the proportion of the involved body parts (e.g., "half of the back"). You can also estimate the percentage of the child's body involved in the burn by using the child's palm. The palm is approximately 1 per cent of the total body surface. Add up the number of palm-sized areas of injured skin to estimate the percentage of the body surface involved (**Figure 11-3**).

Often, health professionals describe the depth of a burn in relation to the thickness of the tissues involved. **Superficial burns** involve only the top part of the skin. The skin is pink, but does not blister. When deeper areas, but not the whole thickness of the skin is

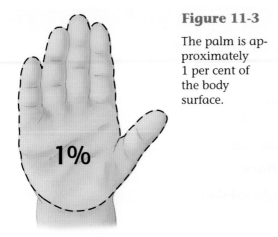

Figure 11-3

The palm is approximately 1 per cent of the body surface.

burned, the injury is called a burn. A **partial-thickness burn** is the type that blisters. A burn that involves the full-thickness of skin may involve deeper tissues under the skin as well. This is the most serious type of burn, called a **full-thickness burn**. A full-thickness burn can damage the full depth of skin, muscle, and nerves (**Figure 11-4**).

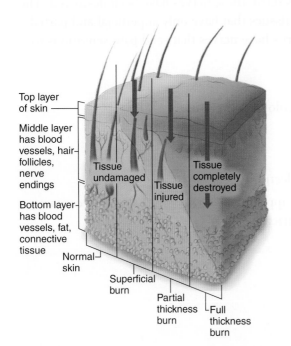

Figure 11-4

Depth of burn injury.

Top layer of skin

Middle layer has blood vessels, hair follicles, nerve endings

Tissue undamaged

Tissue injured

Tissue completely destroyed

Bottom layer has blood vessels, fat, connective tissue

Normal skin

Superficial burn

Partial thickness burn

Full thickness burn

What You Should Look For

Superficial Burn:

- Pink or red skin
- Mild swelling, no blisters
- Mild to moderate pain

Partial-thickness Burn:

- Dark red or bright red skin
- Blisters
- Swelling
- Moderate to severe pain

Full-thickness Burn:

- Red, raw, ash white, black, leathery, or charred skin
- Swelling
- Pain can be severe in the area surrounding a full-thickness burn, although there is little or no pain in the tissues that have a full-thickness burn. In the tissues involved in a full-thickness burn, these nerves have been destroyed. The surrounding tissues that have only superficial and partial-thickness burns have nerves that send pain sensations to the brain.

Chemical Burn:

- A change of colour in the skin
- Pain

Electrical Burn:

- A source of electricity
- Red or white appearance to the skin that was in contact with the electricity

What You Should Do

The Nine Steps in Paediatric First Aid:

1 **Survey the Scene**

Take a brief moment to perform a scene survey to ensure that the scene is safe, to find out who is involved, and to determine what happened.

2 **Hands-off ABCs**

As you approach the child, perform the hands-off ABCs (Appearance, Breathing, and Circulation) to determine if the ambulance service should be called. It should take 15 to 30 seconds or less.

3 **Supervise**

Immediately ensure that any other children near the scene are properly supervised.

4 **Hands-on ABCDEs**

Perform the hands-on ABCDEs (Appearance, Breathing, Circulation, Disability, and Everything else) to determine if the ambulance service should be called and what first aid care is needed.

5 **First Aid Care**

Provide first aid care appropriate to the injury or illness.

6 **Notify**

As soon as possible, notify the child's parent(s) or legal guardian(s).

7 **Debrief**

As soon as possible, talk with the child who received first aid about any concerns he or she may have, and talk with other children who witnessed the injury and first aid procedures.

8 Document

Complete an incident report form.

9 Prevention

Immediately remove or fence off any obvious danger. If this is not possible, report the hazard appropriately and place suitable signage up as an interim measure.

Did You Know

High voltage electricity can jump or arc up to 15 metres. If you find a child near a high voltage source, such as overhead cables, always make sure the source is switched off before approaching.

First Aid Tip

You should provide first aid care for all burns, but the child needs to see a health care professional immediately:
- If the burn is deep, large, or there is blistering
- If the burn is on the face, hands, feet, genital areas, over joints, encircles the upper body, neck, or a limb
- If it is an electrical burn
- If it is a chemical burn
- If smoke or fumes have been inhaled
- If the burn is difficult to manage or help is needed with pain control

First Aid Tip

When cooling any burns on a child, they become at risk to hypothermia, particularly when cooling large areas. Make sure a blanket or piece of clothing is used to keep the child warm, ensuring it does not touch the affected area. Remember, cool the burn, not the child.

What You Should Do

First Aid Care for Burns from Heat Sources, Including Sunburn

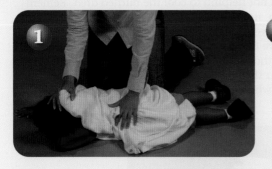

1 Stop the heat injury by removing the child from contact with the source of heat, sunshine, or whatever is causing the burn. If flames are present, smother them by using a blanket or rolling the child on the floor or ground. Prevent the child from running because this fans the flames.

2 Unless a very large part of the body is involved, use cool water right away to take the heat out of the body tissues and reduce the pain in the injured area. You should cool a superficial, partial-thickness, or full-thickness burn even if it involves a large area. If cooling large areas, make sure the child is kept warm with a blanket (avoiding the injured area). Remember to cool the burn, not the child. You should continue to cool the burn until the pain stops or the child receives medical assistance. This approach will avoid chilling the whole body. You should continue to cool a burn, even one that is a full-thickness burn, until the pain stops or the child gets medical care.

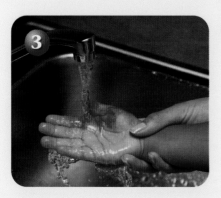

3 To cool a burn, you can place the burned area in a container of cool water or let a gentle (not forceful) flow of cool tap water run over the burned area. Sometimes children will cooperate with this first aid care if they are allowed to play in the cool water with a few toys. If you cannot put the burned area into cool water, (e.g., a burn on the face) cover it with a cold, wet towel, rewetting or replacing the towel every 1 to 2 minutes to keep the towel cool. Another approach is to put a cold pack on top of a wet towel covering the injured area.

First Aid Care for Burns from Heat Sources, Including Sunburn (cont.)

 Prevent chilling of the child from cooling a burn by removing any wet clothing that is not helping to cool the burned area. Remember to cool the burn, not the child. Do not remove clothing that is stuck to the skin. If wet clothing is stuck to skin, cut around the stuck area to remove the wet clothing that is not stuck to the skin. Leave the clothing that is stuck to the skin alone. Then cover unburned areas with a sheet or blankets as needed to keep the child comfortably warm while keeping the burned area cool.

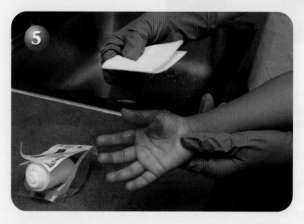

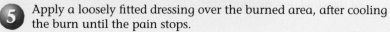 Apply a loosely fitted dressing over the burned area, after cooling the burn until the pain stops.

What You Should Do

First Aid Care for Chemical Burns

1 Stop the injury by removing the child from contact with the chemical.

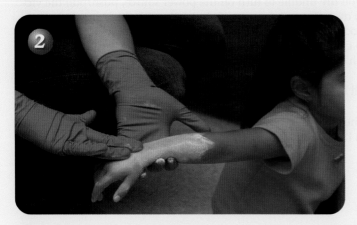

2 Brush off any dry chemical that remains on the skin. Remove constricting items such as jewellery.

3 Call the ambulance service.

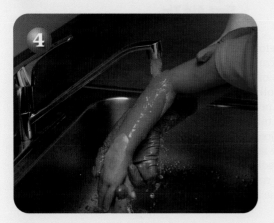

4 Rinse the area of the body that was in contact with the chemical with a continuous gentle flow of fresh water over the entire affected area for 15 to 20 minutes.

What You Should Do

First Aid Care for Electrical Burns

1 Be sure that the child is no longer connected to the source of the electricity. Turn off the power source before approaching the child. If you are unable to turn off the power source, push/pull the victim away from the source of electricity with thick dry cloth or wood stick (broom handle or chair) or a dry towel looped around the child's feet. Never touch the child while he is still in contact with the current or you may also get electrocuted.

2 Call the ambulance service.

3 If the child is unresponsive, follow the steps for difficulty breathing (See Chapter 3).

First Aid Tip

- Always cover ice before putting it on a burn. Direct application of ice to body tissues can damage fragile tissues that remain.
- Do not apply burn ointments, petroleum jelly, margarine, toothpaste or anything other than fresh cool water as first aid care for a burn. A medical professional should prescribe any medications that are used on a burn.
- Keep blisters from breaking if you can. An unbroken blister is a sterile dressing over the injured tissue that helps to prevent infection. When the blister breaks, germs can get into the damaged tissues and grow. After the cooling step is completed, place a loose protective dressing over the blisters to try to keep them from breaking.

Algorithm

First Aid Care for Burns

Remove child from source of burn (heat, chemical, sunshine, electricity)

Call the ambulance service if burn is large or deep, involve face, hands, feet, joints, or genitals, or if smoke or fumes were inhaled.

Cool the burn until the pain stops or the ambulance service arrives. If cooling large areas, make sure the child is kept warm. Remember to cool the burn, not the child.

While cooling the burn area, keep the child warm with clean sheets or blankets

Check Your Knowledge

1. For a child who is outside and appears to have sunburn, you should first:

   a. Remove the child from exposure to sunlight.

   b. Comfort the child.

   c. Put a hat on the child.

   d. Put ice on the sunburn.

2. When blisters form in the area of the burn the person providing first aid should:

   a. Wipe off a sewing needle with alcohol and puncture the blister so the fluid drains out.

   b. Press on the blister to see if the fluid will drain from it.

   c. Wash the blister with soap and water and then cover it with petroleum jelly.

   d. Cover the blister with a loose, protective dressing to try to keep the blister intact.

3. Describe the different between superficial, partial-thickness, and full-thickness burns in relation to the layers of a child's skin.

   _____

   _____

   _____

4. What three factors determine the severity of a burn?

   _____

   _____

   _____

Terms

Burn   An injury to the skin that results from heat, cold, radiation, a chemical, or electrical damage to the body.

Full-thickness burns   Burns that involve the entire thickness of the skin and deeper tissue.

Partial-thickness burns   Burns to the top and middle layer of the skin which make your skin turn red or purple, swell, and blister.

Superficial burns   Burns that involve only the top part of the skin.

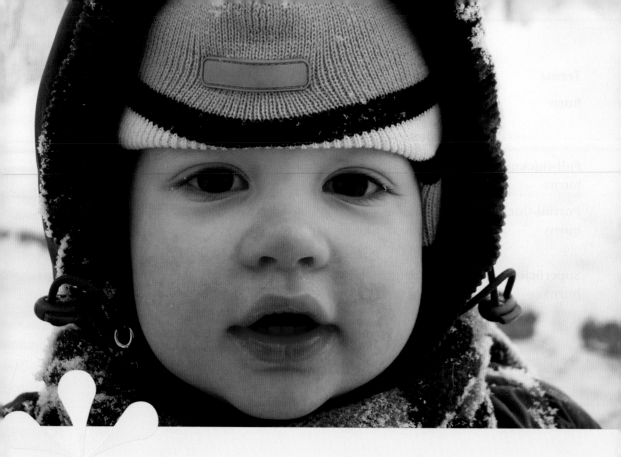

Learning Objectives

The participant will be able to:

- Recognise heat-related injuries (heat stroke, heat exhaustion, heat cramps, dehydration).
- Describe a child who is having a cold-related injury (frostbite, hypothermia).
- Describe appropriate first aid for a child who is having a cold-related injury.
- Identify appropriate first aid for a child who is having a heat-related injury.

Chapter

12

Heat- and Cold- Related Injuries

Heat- and Cold-Related Injuries

Introduction

Infants and small children are more vulnerable to injury from the extremes of heat and cold than adults. Children get chilled and overheated more quickly than adults. Children are also less aware of the dangers from the heat and cold.

Injury from extremes of heat and cold is not only related to temperature but also to factors such as humidity, wind, clothing, and length of exposure. Two terms that help describe the risk of injury from heat and cold are **wind chill** and **heat index.** Wind chill is the difference between the actual temperature and how cold it feels. The wind carries heat away from the body, cooling it more rapidly than would otherwise occur. The heat index is how hot it feels because of humidity and temperature. At higher levels of humidity, it is harder for perspiration to evaporate. Without cooling of the body by evaporation of sweat, it is easier for the body to become overheated.

Heat-Related Illness

What You Should Know

The body produces heat constantly. The body produces more heat during exercise and sometimes during illness. When body temperatures exceed the normal body temperature (37°C), the body has a fever. Normally, in an environment without excessive heat, body temperatures from illness will not exceed 40°C. Temperatures above 40°C can cause permanent harm to the body.

When it is hot, cooling is largely accomplished by the evaporation of sweat. If the air is already humid, sweat does not evaporate quickly, so cooling by sweating becomes less efficient. Some children do not sweat enough to cool themselves as well as other children. Wearing fabrics that trap sweat can restrict cooling.

Usually, the first signs of excess body heat are nausea, headache, and disorientation. If the body temperature does not go down, brain damage and death can occur. The most severe form of heat illness is **heatstroke.** When heatstroke occurs, the body's heat-regulating ability becomes overwhelmed and ceases to function properly, resulting in an inability to sweat and a dangerously high rise in body temperature.

Heatstroke can develop suddenly. An infant or child with heatstroke will have a body temperature of 40°C or higher. Once the ability of the sweat glands to produce sweat is exhausted, the skin may be dry and hot. Often, the skin is flushed. Rapid breathing is present. Usually, confusion or loss of consciousness occurs. Heatstroke is far more common among the elderly and in athletes, but can occur in an active child or in an infant who is overly clothed and insufficiently cooled off.

Heat exhaustion is the result of prolonged exposure to a hot environment, often while actively playing and sweating. Heat exhaustion is largely the result of dehydration from failing to drink a sufficient amount of water to replace fluid that is lost through sweating (**Figure 12-1**). **Heat cramps** are painful muscle spasms, often in the legs. Heat cramps are the result of dehydration in the body caused by insufficient replacement of water lost by sweating.

A child suffering from heat exhaustion will be thirsty and sweating heavily. Pay attention to how often children are urinating during hot conditions and what colour the urine is. If the urine is dark and the child is not urinating at least once every 4 hours, you can prevent dehydration by encouraging the child to drink more often, even if the child only drinks a small amount at a time. A child who has heat exhaustion may feel weak, nauseated, and very tired. There is little or no elevation of the body temperature at this stage of heat illness. The child's tongue and mouth are likely to look dry. Heat cramps may accompany heat exhaustion. A child may complain of muscle cramps, usually in the legs and abdominal muscles.

Did You Know

In the summer of 2003, a severe heat wave occurred in France and other parts of Europe. Over 10,000 people died in France of heatstroke. All ages were involved, but most of the victims were elderly.

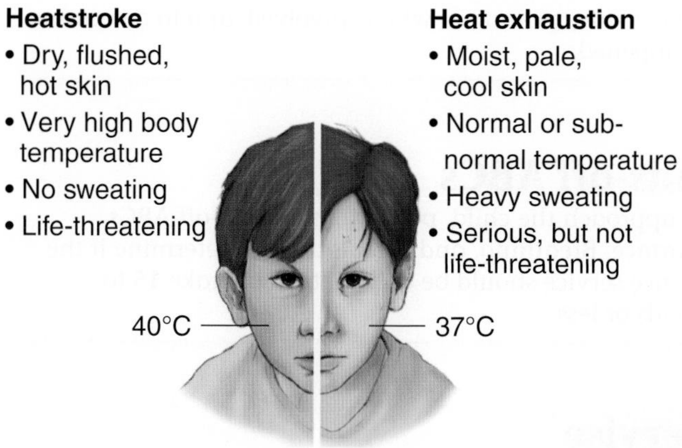

Heatstroke
- Dry, flushed, hot skin
- Very high body temperature
- No sweating
- Life-threatening

Heat exhaustion
- Moist, pale, cool skin
- Normal or sub-normal temperature
- Heavy sweating
- Serious, but not life-threatening

40°C — 37°C

Figure 12-1

Comparison between heat stroke and heat exhaustion.

What You Should Look For

- Heavy sweating for more than a short time, or no sweating when the environment is hot
- Looks and acts ill or more tired than expected; an older child complains of nausea or headache
- Not urinating at least once every 4 hours and not drinking very often when the environment is hot
- Skin is flushed, especially the face
- Disoriented, confused
- Breathing rapidly
- Body temperature is elevated

What You Should Do

The Nine Steps in Paediatric First Aid:

1 Survey the Scene

Take a brief moment to perform a scene survey to ensure that the scene is safe, to find out who is involved, and to determine what happened.

2 Hands-off ABCs

As you approach the child, perform the hands-off ABCs (Appearance, Breathing, and Circulation) to determine if the ambulance service should be called. It should take 15 to 30 seconds or less.

3 Supervise

Immediately ensure that any other children near the scene are properly supervised.

4 Hands-on ABCDEs

Perform the hands-on ABCDEs (Appearance, Breathing, Circulation, Disability, and Everything else) to determine if the ambulance service should be called and what first aid care is needed.

5 First Aid Care

Provide first aid care appropriate to the injury or illness.

6 Notify

As soon as possible, notify the child's parent(s) or legal guardian(s).

7 Debrief

As soon as possible, talk with the child who received first aid about any concerns he or she may have, and talk with other children who witnessed the injury and first aid procedures.

8 Document

Complete an incident report form.

9 Prevention

Immediately remove or fence off any obvious danger. If this is not possible, report the hazard appropriately and place suitable signage up as an interim measure.

What You Should Do

First Aid Care for Heat Exhaustion and Heat Cramps

1 Cool the child immediately and call the ambulance service.

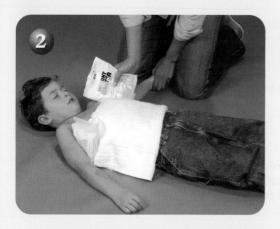

2 Cooling is best accomplished by pouring lots of cool water over the child. If the child tolerates it, put ice packs or ice wrapped in a wet cloth in the armpits and groin of the child. This will cool the blood that goes through the big blood vessels close to the skin in those areas.

What You Should Do

First Aid Care for Heatstroke

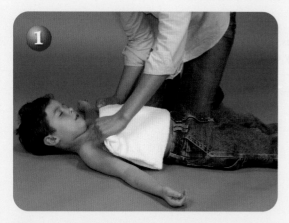

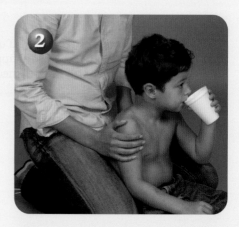

1 Move the child into a cool place. If a cool place is not available, cool the child's body by pouring cool water over the skin or use wet cool cloths. Continue to rinse and reapply cool cloths after they become warmed by contact with the body.

2 Encourage the child to drink of lots of water. The "sports drinks" are not better than water, and water is more readily available.

Cold-Related Injuries

What You Should Know

Hypothermia is a dangerous condition in which, through severe exposure to cold, the core body temperature (the temperature deep within the body) drops below 35°C. Body processes slow at these low temperatures and tissue damage can occur. The cause of hypothermia is prolonged exposure to the cold. Falling into cold water is a common cause, as is being outside too long without proper clothing during cold weather. Body temperatures drop when the body is unable to produce enough heat to compensate for heat loss. The outside temperature does not have to be below freezing for hypothermia to occur.

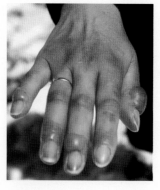

Figure 12-2

Frostbite.

    Frostbite is tissue damage caused by extreme cold (**Figure 12-2**). Ears, face, hands, and feet are especially susceptible because tissues in these areas are thin, exposed, or are far from the body core. **Frostnip** is the most common local cold injury. There is minimal tissue damage and no actual freezing of the tissue.

What You Should Look For

- Body temperature is lower than normal
- Child is sluggish and may be unconscious
- Injured skin with frostnip or frostbite appears cold, pale, and feels numb to the touch
- Injured skin may blister
- When body part is warmed, tissues that have been injured may have more blood in them than usual, may turn pink, or if the damage is severe, may remain pale
- Mild to moderately damaged tissues hurt, tingle, and feel like they are burning

What You Should Do

First Aid Care for Hypothermia

1 Bring the child into a warm place and call the ambulance service. Until you can get to a warm room, bring the child close to someone else's warm body.

2 Strip off the cold wet clothes and replace them with warm dry ones.

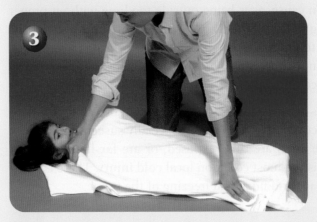

3 Wrap the child in a blanket.

4 If the child is alert, offer them warm drinks and, if possible, carbohydrate-rich foods to give the body energy.

What You Should Do

First Aid Care for Frostbite and Frostnip

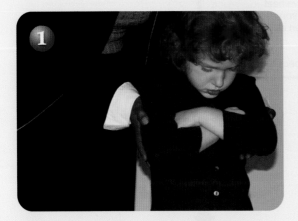

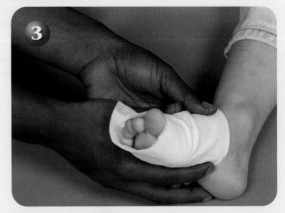

1 Take the child to a warm room and call the ambulance service. Until you can get to a warm room, place cold body parts close to warm body areas. For example, tuck cold hands into the armpits.

2 Remove any wet clothes including shoes and socks, and cover the areas with clean, warm, and dry coverings.

3 Do not break any blisters that may be present, but cover those that have broken with gauze.

4 Allow the cold-injured part to return to normal body temperature slowly.

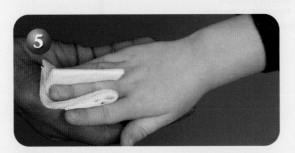

5 If toes or fingers are cold damaged, put dry gauze between the toes or fingers to keep them from rubbing each other.

6 Inform the child's parent(s) or legal guardian(s) that the child may need medical attention.

Algorithm

First Aid Care for Heat-Related Illness

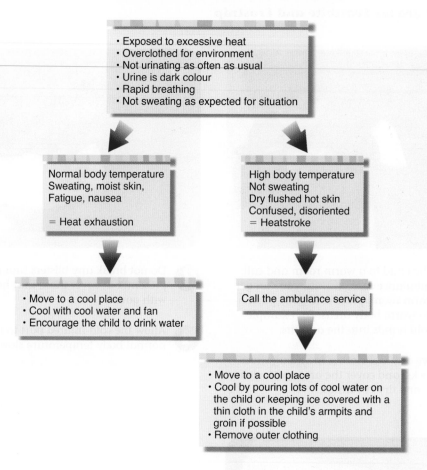

- Exposed to excessive heat
- Overclothed for environment
- Not urinating as often as usual
- Urine is dark colour
- Rapid breathing
- Not sweating as expected for situation

Normal body temperature
Sweating, moist skin,
Fatigue, nausea

= Heat exhaustion

High body temperature
Not sweating
Dry flushed hot skin
Confused, disoriented
= Heatstroke

- Move to a cool place
- Cool with cool water and fan
- Encourage the child to drink water

Call the ambulance service

- Move to a cool place
- Cool by pouring lots of cool water on the child or keeping ice covered with a thin cloth in the child's armpits and groin if possible
- Remove outer clothing

First Aid Care for Hypothermia

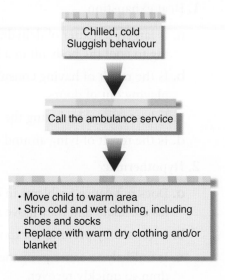

Chilled, cold
Sluggish behaviour

Call the ambulance service

- Move child to warm area
- Strip cold and wet clothing, including shoes and socks
- Replace with warm dry clothing and/or blanket

First Aid Care for Frostbite

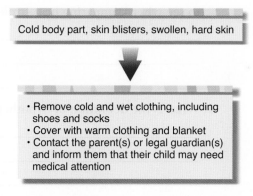

Cold body part, skin blisters, swollen, hard skin

- Remove cold and wet clothing, including shoes and socks
- Cover with warm clothing and blanket
- Contact the parent(s) or legal guardian(s) and inform them that their child may need medical attention

Check Your Knowledge

1. Heat exhaustion:

    a. Is largely a matter of dehydration and inability of sweating to cool the body off in a hot environment.

    b. Is the result of having consumed too much water while playing out of doors.

    c. Is best treated by letting the child rest in the shade.

    d. Is the result of lying around on a hot and humid day.

2. Hypothermia:

    a. Does not cause problems in children because their bodies are small and they move around a lot.

    b. Is caused by prolonged exposure to the cold.

    c. Is unlikely to cause permanent damage, because children so quickly recover.

    d. Causes the child to develop a high fever.

3. What are different signs any symptoms you would expect to see when comparing heat stroke with heat exhaustion?

_____

_____

_____

4. What is the definition of hypothermia?

_____

_____

_____

Terms

Frostbite	Tissue damage caused by extreme cold.
Frostnip	The most common local cold injury. There is minimal tissue damage and no actual freezing of tissue.
Heat cramps	Painful muscle spasms, often in the legs. The result of dehydration in the body caused by insufficient replacement of water lost by sweating.
Heat exhaustion	The result of prolonged exposure to a hot environment, often while actively playing and sweating.
Heat index	The difference between the actual temperature and how hot it feels because of humidity and temperature.
Heatstroke	The body's heat-regulating ability becomes overwhelmed and ceases to function properly, resulting in an inability to sweat and a dangerously high rise in body temperature.
Hypothermia	A dangerous condition in which, through severe exposure to cold, the core body temperature drops below 35°C.
Wind chill	The difference between the actual temperature and how cold it feels.

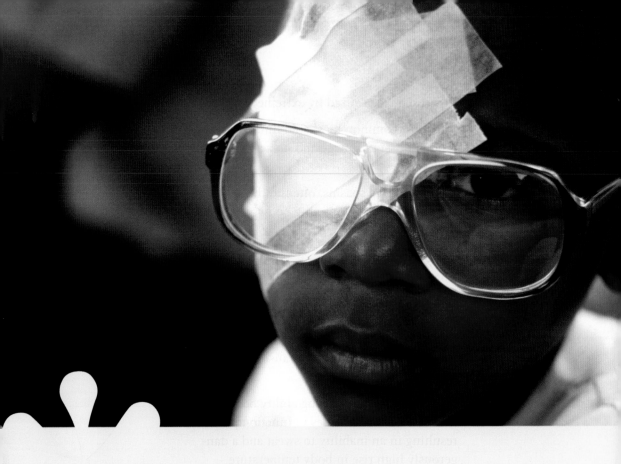

Learning Objectives

The participant will be able to:

- Recognize eye injuries in a child care setting.
- List first aid needed for eye injuries in a child care setting.

Chapter

13

Eye Injuries

Eye Injuries

Introduction

An **eye injury** includes injury to the eye, eyelid, and area around the eye. Common eye injuries result from scratches, cuts, foreign bodies, burns, chemicals, and blows to the eye. The main concern when a child has suffered from an eye injury is possible damage to the child's vision. Eye injuries are the most common and preventable causes of blindness.

What You Should Know

Eye trauma refers to any injury to the eye. Eye trauma occurs often in children and is a common cause of loss of vision. According to the National Society to Prevent Blindness, approximately ⅓ of eye loss in children under 10 years of age is due to trauma to the eye. Activities that are commonly associated with eye trauma include: archery, hockey, darts, BB guns, bicycling, baseball, boxing, basketball, and sports that involve rackets. Fingernails, toys, and chemicals are also common causes of trauma. Each year, toys and home playground equipment cause thousands of injuries to young eyes.

What You Should Look For

- Double vision
- Decrease in vision
- Sensitivity to light
- Redness or swelling
- Pain when moving the eye in any direction
- Blood in the eye (haemorrhage)
- Dizziness
- Numbness
- Inability to open eye after trauma

Any of the above symptoms indicate that this child should receive immediate medical attention.

What You Should Do

The Nine Steps in Paediatric First Aid:

1 Survey the Scene

Take a brief moment to perform a scene survey to ensure that the scene is safe, to find out who is involved, and to determine what happened.

2 Hands-off ABCs

As you approach the child, perform the hands-off ABCs (Appearance, Breathing, and Circulation) to determine if the ambulance service should be called. It should take 15 to 30 seconds or less.

3 Supervise

Immediately ensure that any other children near the scene are properly supervised.

4 Hands-on ABCDEs

Perform the hands-on ABCDEs (Appearance, Breathing, Circulation, Disability, and Everything else) to determine if the ambulance service should be called and what first aid care is needed.

5 First Aid Care

Provide first aid care appropriate to the injury or illness.

6 Notify

As soon as possible, notify the child's parent(s) or legal guardian(s).

7 Debrief

As soon as possible, talk with the child who received first aid about any concerns he or she may have, and talk with other children who witnessed the injury and first aid procedures.

8 Document

Complete an incident report form.

9 Prevention

Immediately remove or fence off any obvious danger. If this is not possible, report the hazard appropriately and place suitable signage up as an interim measure.

What You Should Do

First Aid Care for Chemical Injury to the Eye

1 Wear disposable gloves and immediately flush the chemical from the eye with lukewarm water.

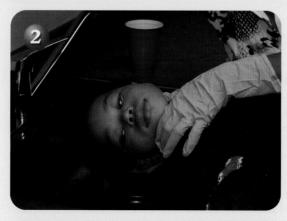

2 Position the head over a sink with the injured eye down to prevent the rinse water from contaminating the other eye.

3 Hold the injured eye open with your fingers and flush with water for 15 minutes.

4 Rinse from the inside of the eye toward the outside. You may need to securely hold the child still.

5 Seek immediate medical advice, either call the ambulance service or take the child to the nearest Accident and Emergency (A&E) department.

6 Inform the child's parent(s) or legal guardian(s) that the child should be seen by a health care professional.

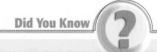

Did You Know

Chemicals get into children's eyes most commonly from products in spray bottles, such as household cleaners and pesticides. A chemical burn to the eye requires immediate first aid treatment to prevent damage to the **cornea,** the transparent outer covering of the eyeball. Eye damage can occur swiftly—in less than 5 minutes. Certain chemical agents can cause rapid and severe damage. The eye may not appear red, but vision may be threatened.

First Aid Tip

Whilst foreign bodies in the eye can often be easily removed, anything stuck in a child's ear should be removed by a health care professional, either at a general practitioner surgery, a minor injuries unit, walk-in centre, or at the nearest A&E department. Foreign bodies lodged in the nose can often be blown out. Encourage the child to blow their nose whilst occluding the unaffected nostril. Try this three times; if it is not cleared, take the child to a minor injuries unit, walk-in centre, or the nearest A&E department. Do not try and fish the object out as this may only push the object further into the nose.

What You Should Do

First Aid Care for Penetrating Injury to the Eye

 Call the ambulance service.

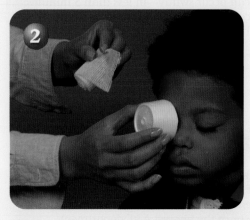

2 Penetrating eye injuries generally include lacerations, or open wounds in the eye. Attempt to cover the injured eye with an eye shield, paper cup, or even cardboard folded into a cone. If the child strongly resists covering the eye, do not insist.

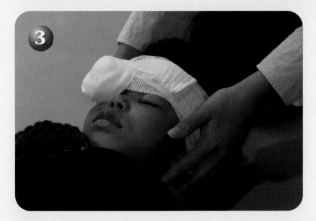

3 Keep the child as quiet as possible. The best position is for the child to lie still and be flat on his back, but do not force the child to lie in this position if he resists. Never attempt to remove a foreign object penetrating the eye, since this may cause more damage than the initial injury. Never apply pressure to the eye. Do not apply medication or preparations.

What You Should Do

First Aid Care for Foreign Object in the Eye

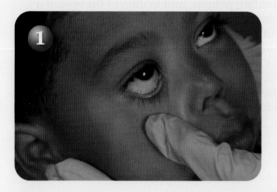

1 A foreign body can be any material (e.g., dust, sand, paint) which gets into the eye. Wear disposable gloves and pull down the child's lower eyelid to look at the inner surface while the child looks up. A speck of dirt can usually be removed with a clean wet gauze or handkerchief.

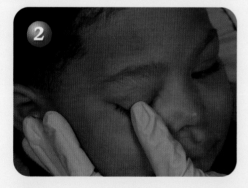

2 Gently grasp the upper lid and pull it out and down over the lower eyelid. Tears that occur when you pull the upper lid over the lower lid may help dislodge the object.

3 If the object remains, flush the eye with water. Position the head over a sink, injured eye down. Hold the eye open with your fingers and use an unbreakable cup to rinse from the inside (nose side) of the eye toward the outside (ear side) of the eye. Do not apply medication.

4 The child should be examined by a health care professional if the eye continues to tear or be red or painful. The foreign body might have scratched the cornea, and this injury can only be confirmed by a professional with a special dye and medical equipment.

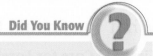

Did You Know

Eye lashes, dirt, insects, and bits of sand are foreign objects that commonly cause discomfort, redness, and tearing of the eyes. If a child has a foreign object in the eye, rubbing the eye can scratch the cornea. A scratch of the cornea is commonly called a **corneal abrasion.** A corneal abrasion is very painful, and can lead to a threatening infection. Covering an injured eye may reduce some of the pain, but it will not heal the injury. Do not force the child to accept a cover since this may cause further injury to the eye if there is something under the eyelid or stuck in the eye.

What You Should Do

First Aid Care for Cut on the Eye or Lid

1 Keep the child in a seated position.

2 Wear disposable gloves.

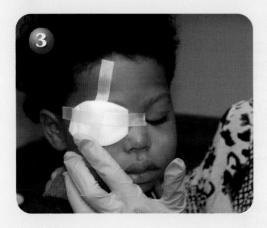

3 If the child will tolerate it, cover the injured eye with a gauze pad and bandage loosely. Do not attempt to flush the eye with water or apply pressure to the injured eyelid. Do not apply medication.

4 Inform the child's parent(s) or legal guardian(s) that the child should be seen by a health care professional.

What You Should Do

First Aid Care for Blow to the Eye

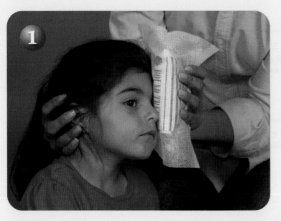

1 Gently place ice pack or a cold pack wrapped in a wet cloth on the injured eye for 10 to 15 minutes to control swelling and reduce pain.

2 A black eye, redness, pain, or blurred vision might indicate internal eye damage or swelling, and the child should be seen by a health care professional as soon as possible. Do not apply medication.

Algorithm

First Aid Care for Chemical in the Eye

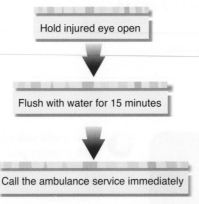

Hold injured eye open

⬇

Flush with water for 15 minutes

⬇

Call the ambulance service immediately

First Aid Care for Penetrating Object in the Eye

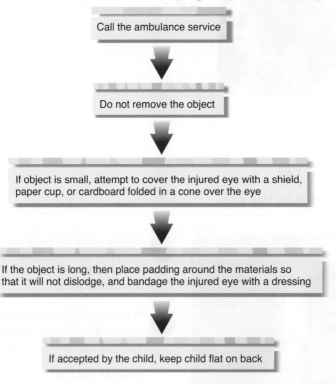

Call the ambulance service

⬇

Do not remove the object

⬇

If object is small, attempt to cover the injured eye with a shield, paper cup, or cardboard folded in a cone over the eye

⬇

If the object is long, then place padding around the materials so that it will not dislodge, and bandage the injured eye with a dressing

⬇

If accepted by the child, keep child flat on back

First Aid Care for a Foreign Object in the Eye

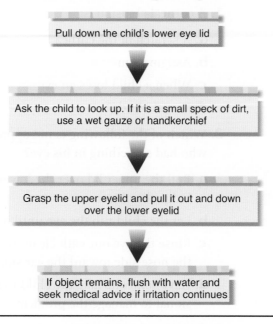

Pull down the child's lower eye lid

Ask the child to look up. If it is a small speck of dirt, use a wet gauze or handkerchief

Grasp the upper eyelid and pull it out and down over the lower eyelid

If object remains, flush with water and seek medical advice if irritation continues

First Aid Care for a Cut on the Eye

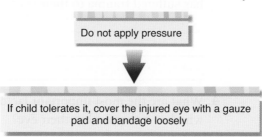

Do not apply pressure

If child tolerates it, cover the injured eye with a gauze pad and bandage loosely

Check Your Knowledge

1. A corneal abrasion is:

    a. A scratch of the cornea

    b. Astigmatism

    c. When a child loses an eye

    d. Partial blindness

2. Which of the following is <u>not appropriate</u> care for a child who had something in his eye?

    a. Pull the upper lid over the lower lid so the tears can dislodge the object

    b. Let the child rub the eye until it feels better

    c. Rinse the eye out with clean, running tap water, from the nose side toward the ear side of the eye

    d. Have someone take the child to a health care professional to manage the problem

3. What are the main signs and symptoms for a child who has suffered trauma to their eye?

_____

_____

_____

4. What are the most important factors when treating a child who has a chemical in their eye?

_____

_____

_____

Terms

Cornea	The transparent outer covering of the eyeball.
Corneal abrasion	A scratch of the cornea.
Eye injury	Injury to the eye, eyelid, and area around the eye.
Eye trauma	Any injury to the eye.

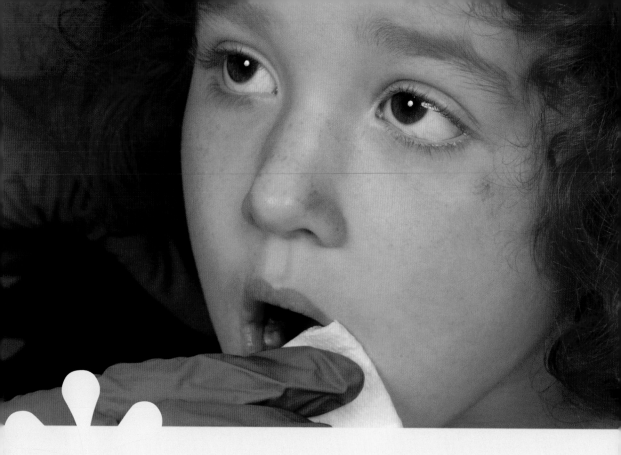

Learning Objectives

The participant will be able to:

- Recognise when a tooth has been knocked out.
- Describe first aid for a knocked-out tooth.
- Describe first aid for a toothache.
- Recognise when a child has a bite to the tongue or lips.
- Describe first aid for a bite to the tongue or lips.

Chapter

14 Oral Injuries

Teeth

Introduction

Most children start getting teeth at approximately 6 months of age, and will have a full set of primary, or "baby", teeth by 3 years of age. **Primary teeth** serve a number of purposes. They are involved in speech development, they help maintain good nutrition by allowing the child to chew properly, and they act as space savers for **permanent teeth**. When a child is about 6 years old, his jaw will begin to grow to make room for permanent, or "adult", teeth. From the ages of 6 to 12 years, children will lose primary teeth and permanent teeth will replace them.

What You Should Know

A permanent tooth that is knocked out is a dental emergency that needs immediate first aid. A child with a knocked-out tooth needs to be seen by a dentist as soon as possible. A permanent tooth that is knocked out should be placed back into the socket. This gives the tooth a greater chance of survival. Primary, or baby, teeth should not be reinserted. If a primary tooth is knocked out, the child needs first aid care for any gum injuries and should be seen by a dentist.

What You Should Look For

- A missing tooth in the child's mouth
- Bleeding from the mouth
- Visibly upset child

Did You Know

A tooth that has been knocked out will start to die within 15 to 30 minutes. Relocating it as soon as possible is imperative.

What You Should Do

The Nine Steps in Paediatric First Aid:

1 Survey the Scene

Take a brief moment to perform a scene survey to ensure that the scene is safe, to find out who is involved, and to determine what happened.

2 Hands-off ABCs

As you approach the child, perform the hands-off ABCs (Appearance, Breathing, and Circulation) to determine if the ambulance service should be called. It should take 15 to 30 seconds or less.

3 Supervise

Immediately ensure that any other children near the scene are properly supervised.

4 Hands-on ABCDEs

Perform the hands-on ABCDEs (Appearance, Breathing, Circulation, Disability, and Everything else) to determine if the ambulance service should be called and what first aid care is needed.

5 First Aid Care

Provide first aid care appropriate to the injury or illness.

6 Notify

As soon as possible, notify the child's parent(s) or legal guardian(s).

7 Debrief

As soon as possible, talk with the child who received first aid about any concerns he or she may have, and talk with other children who witnessed the injury and first aid procedures.

8 Document

Complete an incident report form.

9 Prevention

Immediately remove or fence off any obvious danger. If this is not possible, report the hazard appropriately and place suitable signage up as an interim measure.

What You Should Do

First Aid Care for Knocked Out Permanent Tooth

1 Position the child so blood does not compromise his airway.

2 Follow Standard Precautions and control any bleeding.

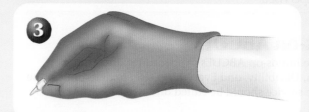

3 Attempt to find the tooth. If you find the tooth, do not handle it by the roots.

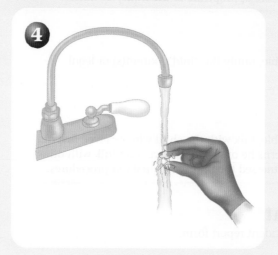

4 If the tooth is dirty, rinse it gently with water. Do not scrub or use antiseptic on the tooth.

First Aid Care for Knocked Out Permanent Tooth (cont.)

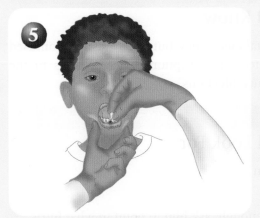

5 Gently place the tooth back in the socket. If the child is able to assist, ask him to hold the tooth in place with a finger or tissue. Do not attempt to reinsert a primary/baby tooth.

6 If the child is upset or resists, or if reinserting the tooth is not possible, place the tooth in a glass of milk. If milk is not available, wrap the tooth in a cold wet cloth.

7 Notify the parent(s) or legal guardian(s) and inform them that the child should be seen by a dentist or health care professional. For best results, the child should be seen by a dentist within 1 hour of the time the tooth was knocked out.

First Aid Tip

If you are unable to locate a knocked-out tooth, it is still important to have the child seen by a dentist as soon as possible because the tooth may be knocked up into the gums. This is true regardless of whether the tooth is a primary or permanent tooth.

Toothache

What You Should Know

Toothache may be a dental emergency, but it may also be confused with discomfort associated with eruption of teeth, sores in the mouth, earaches, and sinus infections.

What You Should Look For

- Complaints of pain
- Drooling
- If the child is old enough, ask him to point to what hurts and have him indicate which tooth hurts.

What You Should Do

First Aid Care for Toothaches

1 Follow Standard Precautions.

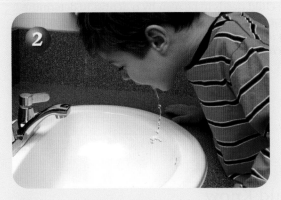

2 Have the child rinse his mouth with warm water.

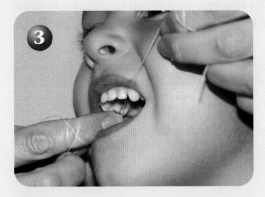

3 Use dental floss to remove any food that might be caught between the teeth.

4 Look for swelling or a "pimple" around the tooth, which may indicate a dental abscess.

5 See if the tooth is loose.

6 Notify the parent(s) or legal guardian(s) and inform them that the child has a toothache and may need to be seen by a dentist or health care professional.

First Aid Tip

If a child complains of a toothache, a health care professional may be able to identify a problem such as an infection or mouth sores that are giving the child the sensation of a toothache. If these are not the problem, the child needs to be seen by a dentist to determine the cause of the discomfort and to prescribe the proper treatment. If there is any swelling in the mouth or on the face, the child needs to be seen by a health care professional or dentist as soon as possible.

Bites

What You Should Know

Children often bite their lips or tongues while eating or during a fall. A bite to the tongue or lips may be difficult to evaluate because the large amount of bleeding may disguise the true size of the injury.

What to Look For

- A hole in the lip or tongue that is the size and shape of a tooth mark
- Bleeding

What Should You Do

First Aid Care for Bites to the Tongue or Lips

1 Follow Standard Precautions.

2 Have the child rinse with water so that the site of injury can be identified.

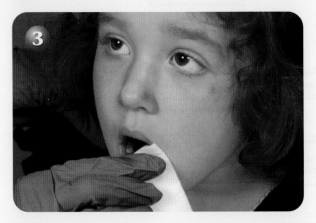

3 Apply pressure with a piece of gauze or cloth to stop the bleeding.

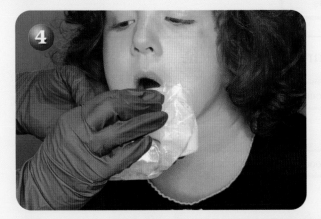

4 Apply ice or a cold pack wrapped in cloth or towel if there is any swelling.

5 Injuries that extend through the lip or that cut across the edge of the tongue should be seen by a health care professional. These injuries may need stitches.

Algorithm

First Aid Care for a Knocked Out Tooth

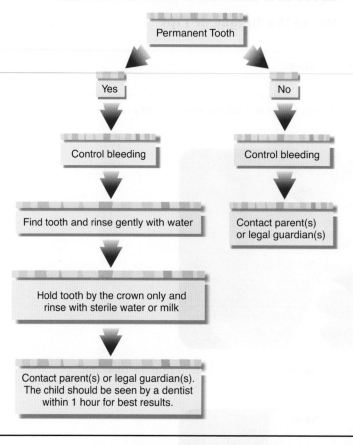

Permanent Tooth

Yes → Control bleeding → Find tooth and rinse gently with water → Hold tooth by the crown only and rinse with sterile water or milk → Contact parent(s) or legal guardian(s). The child should be seen by a dentist within 1 hour for best results.

No → Control bleeding → Contact parent(s) or legal guardian(s)

First Aid Care for a Toothache

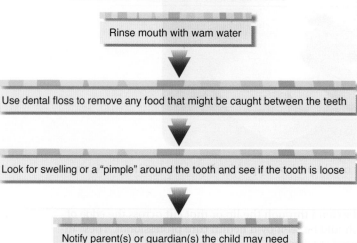

Rinse mouth with wam water

Use dental floss to remove any food that might be caught between the teeth

Look for swelling or a "pimple" around the tooth and see if the tooth is loose

Notify parent(s) or guardian(s) the child may need to be seen by a dentist or health care professional

First Aid Care for Lip and Tongue Bites

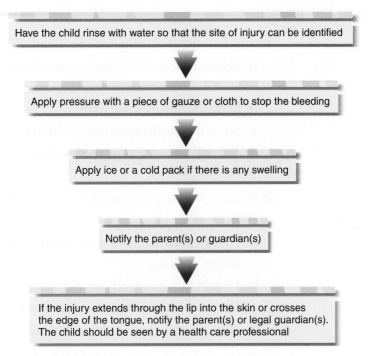

Have the child rinse with water so that the site of injury can be identified

Apply pressure with a piece of gauze or cloth to stop the bleeding

Apply ice or a cold pack if there is any swelling

Notify the parent(s) or guardian(s)

If the injury extends through the lip into the skin or crosses the edge of the tongue, notify the parent(s) or legal guardian(s). The child should be seen by a health care professional

Check Your Knowledge

Circle the letter next to the response that is the best answer to each question.

1. If a child has had a tooth knocked out, you should:

   a. Reinsert the tooth, regardless of whether it is a permanent tooth or primary tooth

   b. Reinsert only primary teeth

   c. Scrub the tooth and bring the child to the dentist

   d. Attempt to reinsert the tooth only if it is a permanent tooth

2. Primary teeth are important for all of the following reasons, except:

   a. They help to maintain good nutrition by enabling proper chewing

   b. They help with speech development

   c. They act as space savers for permanent teeth

   d. They prevent children from choking

3. What actions should you take for a child with a toothache?

   _____

   _____

   _____

4. What actions should you take for a child who has bitten their lip whilst playing?

   _____

   _____

   _____

Terms

Permanent teeth   Teeth that develop at about 6 years of age to replace primary teeth. By age 21, usually all 32 of the permanent teeth have erupted.

Primary teeth   Also known as baby teeth, primary teeth usually begin to grow at about 6 months of age. Most children have a full set of primary teeth at about age 3.

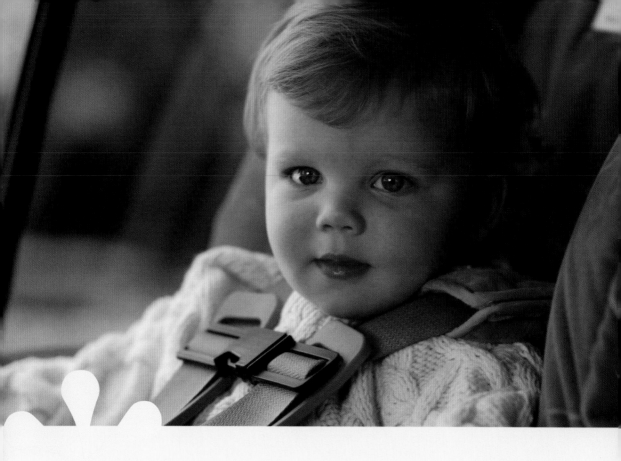

Chapter
15 Prevention

Prevention

Introduction

As a carer or teacher, you have the important task of caring and nurturing for young children. In addition to the nurturing aspects of your work, you must also think constantly about the safety of the children. Because children cannot always make judgements about their own health and safety, they tend to be at a greater risk for injuries, such as burns, falls, choking, and poisoning (**Figure 15-1**). Unintentional injuries are often referred to as accidents because they occur unexpectedly and seem uncontrollable. However, most injuries are avoidable if a few simple steps are practiced consistently. **Prevention** is the use of safety measures to reduce risk. In a child care setting, carers and teachers should seek to reduce the risk of significant injury or illness to children in their care.

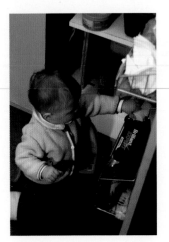

Figure 15-1

Because children cannot always make judgements about their own health and safety, they tend to be at a greater risk for injuries, such as burns, falls, choking, and poisoning.

What You Should Know

Children learn about their environment by exploring; particularly with their senses of taste and touch. Being aware of the dangers in a child's environment and knowing how you can make that environment safer are important in preventing childhood injury and illness. As children grow, the hazards they face change because of their advancing capabilities. Children in a child care setting may be at different ages and developmental stages. This can make creating and maintaining a safe environment particularly challenging. A carer or teacher who understands a child's growth and development is invaluable in reducing hazards in the environment with safe, age-appropriate items.

Carers should seek to maintain child-safe play equipment on playgrounds and in classrooms (**Figure 15-2**). The most common locations for injury in the child care setting are indoor and outdoor play areas. According to the Royal Society for the Prevention of Accidents (RoSPA), it is estimated that each year 40,000 injuries to children occur in playgrounds which result in a hospital visit. The majority of accidents are related to falls, either falling from equipment or tripping/falling over. Only a small percentage involve being

Figure 15-2

Carers should seek to maintain child-safe play equipment on playgrounds and in classrooms.

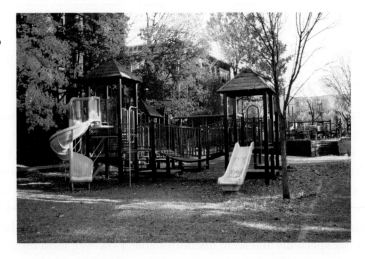

Common Injuries Related to a Child's Developmental Level

Developmental Characteristics	Common Injuries
Infant—Age 0 to 1 year	
Increasing mobility	Burns
Uses mouth to explore objects	Choking
Reaches for and pulls objects	Drowning
Unaware of dangers	Falls
Cannot understand "no"	
Toddler—Age 1 to 2½ years	
Travels in cars	Burns
Masters walking, running, climbing	Choking
Explores almost everything with mouth	Drowning
Begins to imitate behaviours	Falls
Investigates everything within reach	Motor vehicle passenger
Curious about never-before-seen items	and pedestrian injuries
Unaware of most dangers	Poisoning
Impulsive	Suffocation
Preschool-age—Age 2½ to 5 years	
Travels in cars	Burns
Mobility leads to increased	Choking
independence	Drowning
Learns to ride tricycle	Falls
Unaware of many dangers	Motor vehicle passenger
Might favour real tools, gadgets,	and pedestrian injuries
appliances rather than toys	Poisoning
Fascinated with fire	
Imitates adult behaviour	
School-aged—Age 5 years and up	
Travels in cars	Bicycle injuries
Walks alone	Burns
Seeks independence	Falls
Wants to be like peers	Motor vehicle passenger
Likes to be with peers	and pedestrian injuries
Needs increased physical activity	
Dangers do not always seem real	
Increased independence can	
mean less supervision	

struck (ie, by a swing seat). The standards which govern playgrounds are EN1176 for playground equipment and EN1177 for surfacing. The RoSPA website has a comprehensive amount of information relating to playground safety and accident prevention.

What You Should Look For

Identifying potential dangers is an initial step in creating a safe environment. The first thing that you can do to recognise potential danger is to conduct a child's eye-level inspection in every room of the child care facility. For example, look for electrical outlets that do not have protective covers on them to prevent access by children and any cleaning supplies or household products that could be within a child's reach. Check that all hanging cords, table coverings, and lamps are out of reach and cannot be pulled on by a child. Are the medicine cabinets locked and the doors that lead to stairways, outdoors, and storage areas properly secured? Check all indoor and outdoor equipment that is accessible to children. Is the equipment well-maintained and appropriate for the developmental level of the children? Creative use of play areas and thoughtful storage of toys may be required.

Each day before children arrive at the facility, a carer or teacher should take a quick walk around the facility to make sure that the facility is safe and clean. Learning and following the prevention measures outlined in "What You Should Do" will help you to recognise potential dangers in your facility.

What You Should Do

Prevention steps can reduce the likelihood that you will need to use your first aid skills. However, if a first aid emergency occurs, it is important to follow the nine steps of paediatric first aid.

The Nine Steps in Pediatric First Aid:

1 ## Survey the Scene

Take a brief moment to perform a scene survey to ensure that the scene is safe, to find out who is involved, and to determine what happened.

First Aid Tip

It is important that child care providers have, and are prepared to follow, a care plan for any child with a particular health care need. Carers also need access to a telephone and emergency contact numbers for each child in the facility. This should be accessible both in the facility and during any type of off-site trip.

2 Hands-off ABCs

As you approach the child, perform the hands-off ABCs (Appearance, Breathing, and Circulation) to determine if the ambulance service should be called. It should take 15 to 30 seconds or less.

3 Supervise

Immediately ensure that any other children near the scene are properly supervised.

4 Hands-on ABCDEs

Perform the hands-on ABCDEs (Appearance, Breathing, Circulation, Disability, and Everything else) to determine if the ambulance service should be called and what first aid care is needed.

5 First Aid Care

Provide first aid care appropriate to the injury or illness.

6 Notify

As soon as possible, notify the child's parent(s) or legal guardian(s).

7 Debrief

As soon as possible, talk with the child who received first aid about any concerns he or she may have and also talk with other children who have witnessed the injury and first aid procedures.

8 Document

Complete an incident report form.

9 Prevention

Immediately remove or fence off any obvious danger. If this is not possible, report the hazard appropriately and place suitable signage up as an interim measure.

What You Should Do

Prevention of Injuries

- Any stairway, window, balcony, or elevated surface that is used by or accessible to the children in the facility should be properly secured.

- Remove sharp-edged furniture.

- Do not use baby walkers that can move across the floor. A baby may tip the walker over, fall out of it, or fall down stairs and seriously injure his head. Baby walkers let children get to places where they can pull heavy objects or hot food on themselves.

- Do not leave a baby alone on changing tables, beds, sofas, or chairs.

- Lock the doors to any potentially dangerous areas.

- Use gates or doors on stairways and doorways.

- Window latches and window guards reduce the chance of children falling out of windows. Effective latches prevent windows from opening more than 10 centimetres. Latches should be fitted on all upstairs windows and any other window that a child could climb through.

- There is no legal requirement for protective surfacing to be provided on children's playground. It is, however, recommended by safety organisations such as RoSPA. Visit the RoSPA website for information on play area surfacing.

What You Should Do

Prevention of the Spread of Illnesses

Controlling Bleeding (on page 44) details information about Universal and Standard Precautions. To prevent infection and the spread of illness:

- Reduce contact with germs.

- Use barriers, such as non-porous gloves, disposable nappy changing mats, disposable towels for cleaning-up and disinfecting surfaces, non-porous surfaces that can be cleaned and disinfected, and plastic bags to store contaminated articles until they can be thrown away or disinfected.

- Use whatever tools (e.g., paper towels, tissues, rags, and mops) you have to wipe up any spilled body fluid. Try to use disposable tools to minimise the need to do further cleaning and disinfecting. Avoid spreading spilled body fluid around.
- Put all tools (e.g., paper towels, tissues, rags, mops) that you used to wipe up the spill into a plastic-lined receptacle for disposal or to clean and disinfect later.
- Use a detergent to clean all surfaces in contact with the spill, including floors and rugs.
- Rinse cleaned surfaces with water.
- Apply a disinfecting solution, following the manufacturer's instructions on the label.
- Put body fluid contaminated material used to clean and disinfect the surfaces in a plastic bag with a secure tie for disposal.

What You Should Do

Prevention of Choking

- Supervise mealtime.
- Insist that children sit down while eating. Children should never run, walk, play, or lie down with food in their mouths.
- Cut food for infants and young children into pieces no larger than 1 centimetre. Round foods, like hot dogs and grapes, should be cut long ways.
- Encourage children to chew their food well.
- Be aware of older children's actions. Many choking incidents occur when an older child gives a dangerous food, toy, or small object to a younger child.
- The following foods present a potential choking hazard:
  - Carrots, Cheese Sticks, Grapes, Sausages—Should be sliced long way and then cut up because their diameter is approximately the same size of a baby's/toddler's airway.
  - Apples—Should be sliced thinly because bite sizes are solid and can easily lodge in throats.
  - Oranges—Children may not chew the segment sufficiently and the stringy pulp stays in the mouth, whilst the rest is trapped only part way down the throat.

- Steak—Difficult to chew and often not chewed enough while swallowing
- Cheese chunks—Often too large for a little mouth and when chewed will stay as a lump and may become lodged in the throat
- Ice—Often does not melt fast enough to prevent choking
- Crisps—Often do not soften enough and will scratch the soft lining of the mouth and throat causing discomfort and bleeding

- Avoid toys with small parts and keep other small household items out of the reach of infants and young children.
- Follow the age recommendations on toy packages. Age guidelines reflect the safety of a toy based on any possible choking hazard as well as the child's physical and mental abilities at various ages.
- Check under furniture and between cushions for small items that children could find and put in their mouths.
- Other items that can be choking hazards and should be kept away from infants and young children, include:
  - Balloons
  - Coins
  - Marbles
  - Toys with small parts
  - Toys that can be compressed to fit entirely into a child's mouth
  - Small balls
  - Pen tops
  - Small button-type batteries

What You Should Do

Prevention of Burns

- The water temperature and all hot surfaces accessible to children at the facility should not exceed 43°C.
- Keep cribs, cots, and beds at a safe distance from radiators and electrical outlets.

- Cover outlets with special child-resistant face plates or other safety devices. Plastic plug covers can be a choking hazard if loose-fitting or when removed to use the outlet.
- Do not allow electrical cords to dangle over the edge of countertops.
- Regularly check for frayed or damaged electrical cords.
- Do not use extension cords around infants and toddlers. A child can be electrocuted by biting through a live electric cord.
- Do not run electric cords under rugs in areas of heavy traffic.
- Do not overload electrical circuits.
- Teach children that fire burns.
- Keep matches and lighters out of the reach of children.
- All smoke detectors should be tested and working properly.
- Have a fire escape plan with a designated place for all the children and adults to go. Hold practice fire drills regularly.
- Fire extinguishers should be kept in accessible locations.

What You Should Do

Prevention of Bites and Stings

- When walking in tall grasses, woods, or fields, children's arms and legs should be covered. If possible, tuck trousers into socks and long-sleeved shirts at the waist and have the children wear trainers instead of sandals.
- Stay on trails whenever possible.
- Check children's skin after playing in these areas. Pay special attention to the folds of the skin, the scalp, and the back of the neck. Removing a tick within the first 24 hours greatly reduces the risk of infection.
- Spray insect repellent only when outdoors, use sparingly, and wash hands after applying. Never apply insect repellent to the face, to an open wound, or cut, or to the hands or arms of a child who is likely to put sprayed skin in his mouth.
- Report any insect nests or hives that pose a risk to the children around the facility to the appropriate personnel for removal.

- Check for nests in other locations where children play such as in old tree stumps or playground equipment.
- Avoid rubbish bins and dumpsters.
- When eating outdoors, be aware that many foods attract insects, especially: tuna, peanut butter and jam sandwiches, watermelon, sweetened beverages, and ice cream.

What You Should Do

Prevention of Poisoning

- Limit use of toxic substances as much as possible. For pest control, use the approach that involves sealing up openings that allow pests to enter, putting food in pest-resistant containers, and selecting least-toxic pest control chemicals.
- Eliminate careless storage of poisonous substances. Keep all chemical substances out of reach of children, including household products. Store products in locked cabinets or on high, secure shelves.
- Lock medicine cabinets.
- Avoid interruptions when using a poisonous product.
- Do not store household products with food; the differences between them may not be apparent to a young child.
- Whenever possible, use products with child-resistant safety caps. Remember that, although these are much safer than standard containers, they are not completely childproof. Children watch and imitate adult behaviour, and some children can master the skill of opening the lids. Also, if the lids are not completely closed, they will not be child resistant.
- Keep products in their original, labelled containers. If a poisonous substance is swallowed, correct identification is critical for proper treatment. Do not reuse empty containers such as juice bottles to store chemicals.
- Remember that non-prescription medicines can be just as dangerous as prescription medicines.
- Give prescription medicine only to the child for whom it is intended. What can help one child can harm another.

- Check the medicine label for the dosage each time you administer medication. Use a dose-measuring cup or spoon. More is not better when giving medicine.

- Never call medicine "sweeties".

- In areas accessible to children, identify and remove indoor and outdoor plants at your centre that may be toxic if eaten.

What You Should Do

Prevention of Heat- and Cold-Related Injuries

Heat

- Encourage children to drink cool water frequently.

- Avoid vigorous physical activity during the midday hours when temperatures are usually the highest.

- Encourage parent(s) and legal guardian(s) to dress children in lightweight and loose-fitting, sun-protective clothing in hot weather.

- Never leave a child in a closed vehicle without an adult in the vehicle to directly supervise the child.

- Ensure parents apply the correct factor sun block to their child prior to arriving at the facility on sunny days where outdoor play is planned.

Cold

- Wearing dry mittens, hats, insulated and water-repellent boots and snow pants, and other attire may help to prevent cold injuries.

- Bring a child indoors immediately if he complains of a cold, numb, tingling, or painful area on the body.

What You Should Do

Prevention of Sudden Infant Death Syndrome (SIDS)

Sudden Infant Death Syndrome (SIDS) is described as an unexplained death in infants under 1 year of age. The death is not attributed to any medical condition or external factor, such as abuse or neglect, but is an unexplainable condition with no known preventable causes.

Recommendations to reduce the risk of SIDS are:

- Place infants on their backs when sleeping; utilise a device specially designed to keep babies from rolling over onto their stomachs.
- Do not smoke around or take infants to smoky establishments.
- Avoid overheating the baby with blankets or heaters.

It is important to remember that if the infant is warm and not breathing rescue attempts should not be delayed. Do not waste time, begin rescue breathing immediately, then call the ambulance service.

What You Should Do

Prevention of Other Injuries

Think ahead whenever possible. Consider what could happen if a child was able to get to whatever is in the environment. While making the environment risk-free is not possible, the goal is to avoid situations that are likely to lead to serious injury.

What You Should Do

In Case of a Catastrophic Emergency

- There should be at least one readily available first aid kit wherever children are in care. This includes one for field trips and outings away from the facility and one to remain at the facility. A first aid kit should also be kept in each vehicle that is used to transport children to and from child care. The first aid kits should ideally contain:
  - Disposable nonporous gloves
  - Scissors
  - Tweezers
  - A digital thermometer
  - Adhesive tape
  - Sterile gauze pads

- Conforming bandages
- Triangular bandages
- Safety pins
- Eye dressing
- Pen/pencil and notepad
- Cold pack
- Field dressings
- Plasters
- Plastic bags for cloths, gauze, and other materials used in handling bodily fluids
- Any emergency medications and medical information needed for children with particular health needs
- List of emergency phone numbers and phone numbers for parents and legal guardians

Reporting Accidents and Record Keeping

Schools, nurseries, and child care settings should keep a record of any first aid treatment given. This should include:

- Date, time, and place of incident
- Name (and class) of the injured or ill child
- Details of the injury/illness and what first aid was given
- What happened to the child immediately afterwards (i.e., went home, went back to class, went to hospital)
- Name and signature of the first aider or person dealing with the incident

The information in the record book can:

- Help the school or child care centre identify accident trends and possible areas for improvement in the control of health and safety risks
- Be used for reference in future first aid needs assessments
- Be helpful for insurance and investigative purposes

In an emergency, the teacher or carer in charge should have procedures for contacting the child's parent, guardian, and named contact as soon as possible. It is also good practice to report all serious or significant incidents to the parents by sending a letter home with the child or telephoning the parents.

Check Your Knowledge

1. Prevention:

   a. Is the use of safety measures to minimize risk.

   b. Teaches people how to care for an open wound.

   c. Means there is no longer any risks in the environment.

   d. Stops any accidents from occurring.

2. Barriers that are used to prevent the spread of infection and the spread of illness, include all of the following except:

   a. Non-porous gloves

   b. Disposable towels

   c. Plastic bags

   d. Ointment

3. List types of food that may be considered a choking hazard to young children. Describe how you could prepare the foods to make them safer for young children.

   _____

   _____

   _____

4. List the safety measures within a classroom you can take to help ensure a safe environment.

   _____

   _____

Terms

Prevention   The use of safety measures to minimise
                       potential risk.

Appendices

A: Common Childhood Illnesses

B: Immunisations

C: Infection Control in Schools and Child Care

D: First Aid Kit Contents

Common Childhood Illnesses

Asthma

What You Should Know

Asthma is a condition where the small airways in the lower lungs become inflamed and swell, thus becoming much narrower. This reduces the amount of air that can go in and out of the lungs. Over a million children in the UK have asthma, many of whom will grow out of the condition during later childhood.

Usually a known trigger starts the inflammation and swelling and causes an asthma attack. Common triggers are house dust mites, animal fur, smoke, pollen, and cold air. However, there are many other known and unknown triggers.

The symptoms range from mild to life threatening and vary from child to child. More often than not, with prompt recognition and treatment, the attack is potentially reversible.

What You Should Look For

- Breathlessness
- Inability to complete a sentence when talking

- Wheezing noise when breathing
- Tight chest
- Sitting upright and leaning forward trying to breathe
- Blue lips and nail beds

What You Should Do

Carers and parents should

1. Any child who is exhibiting signs of an asthma attack should receive prompt medical attention. The symptoms can often worsen quicker in a child than in an adult.

2. If a child has a known trigger, ensure that as far as reasonably practicable, the child is kept away from the potential source.

3. Attempt to keep the child calm whilst the ambulance service is responding.

Carers should

1. If a child who is a known asthmatic is demonstrating any of the above symptoms, you should help them locate their medication and encourage them whilst they self-administer. Occasionally, a child may require assistance in assembling a spacer unit for example.

2. Carefully monitor the child when starting a cold or cough, quite often these may exaggerate other symptoms. Have a low threshold for contacting a health care professional when a child is starting to show any signs of breathing difficulty.

3. Make sure that sufficient inhalers and medications are always accessible to the child and that they are in date.

Parent should

1. Follow carer's recommendations.

Child May Return to School or Child Care . . .

There is no reason for a child to be kept at home from school or child care, as long as they feel confident to attend and they have the correct medication with them. Ensure that they have the appropriate amount of medication and that it is in date.

Constipation

What You Should Know

Constipation is defined as hard stools that cause painful elimination. It can be caused by a diet low in fibre and inadequate fluid intake. Sometimes it may result from postponing or resisting the urge to eliminate. Everyone's bowel habits differ. Some go to the toilet more than once a day, whereas other may go once every four days.

What You Should Look For

- Many days without normal bowel movements
- Hard stools that are difficult or painful to pass, or stools that are unusually large or hard to flush down the toilet
- Abdominal pain (stomachaches, cramping, nausea)
- Rectal bleeding from tears called fissures
- Faecal soiling of underwear in a child who has learned to use the toilet
- Poor appetite
- Lack of energy
- Irritable, angry, unhappy
- Foul smelling wind, faeces
- Decreased appetite

What You Should Do

Carers and parents should

1. Encourage the child to drink enough clear fluids to keep the child's urine pale coloured.

2. Encourage the child to eat foods that contain fibre and have a tendency to soften the stool, such as whole-grain products, peaches, prunes, grapes, raisins, plums, melons, carrots, celery, and lettuce.

3. Reduce intake of foods that bind, such as milk, hard cheese, cottage cheese, bananas, apples, apple sauce, and white-flour baked goods.

4. Encourage regular toileting at times when typically a child might need to pass a stool. For most people, the urge to have a bowel movement comes after eating or exercising.

Carers should

Notify parents.

Parents should

1. Work with the child's carer to set regular times for the child to have a relaxed opportunity to use the toilet when the child is most likely to feel the urge to have a bowel movement—usually after meals or after exercise.

2. Call child's health care professional if problem persists for several weeks, or sooner if the child develops vomiting or a large abdomen (belly).

Child May Return to School or Child Care . . .

The child need not be excluded from school or child care.

Coughing

What You Should Know

Coughing is a symptom of an irritation anywhere within the respiratory tract. It often accompanies a viral infection such as a cold. Also, coughing may be caused by an ear infection, allergy, asthma, croup, or infection in any part of the body involved in breathing.

What You Should Look For

- Sore throat
- Dry or wet cough
- Throat irritation
- Hoarse voice, barking cough

What You Should Do

Carers and parents should

1. Teach children to cover their mouths when coughing with a disposable facial tissue if possible or with a shoulder if no facial tissue is available in time.

2. Wash hands thoroughly and often.

3. Watch for difficulty breathing.

Carers should

Notify parents.

Parents should

1. Follow carer recommendations.

2. Notify child's health care professional if child develops a fever, has trouble catching his or her breath, or if cough persists for longer than 1 week.

Child May Return to School or Child Care . . .

Child need not be excluded from school or child care unless the cough is severe or the child has difficulty breathing.

A Possible Cause of Coughing: Croup

What You Should Know

Croup is a viral infection that affects the voice box and the upper airway. It is normally caught through droplets of the virus in the air. Whilst there are many different viruses that may cause croup, it can also be caused by bacteria.

Most commonly, croup affects younger children between the ages of 6 months and 6 years old. Older children who suffer with asthma may also get croup.

Croup is characterised by swelling to the airway, making it difficult for the child to breathe. In some cases, the swelling is so severe that the child needs urgent medical attention. Classically, they will have a "bark-like" cough, caused by swelling to the vocal chords.

What You Should Look For

Croup is most likely to occur in the winter months, with the early symptoms being very similar to having a cold. As the infection develops, symptoms include:

- Bark-like cough
- Croaky voice
- Rasping sound when breathing out

Often these symptoms get worse at night. In some cases, the infection and swelling is so severe that the child will struggle to breathe properly. In these situations, immediate medical attention is required.

What You Should Do

Carers and parents should

1. Teach children to cover their mouths when coughing with a disposable tissue.

2. Monitor children for breathing difficulties and summon assistance accordingly.

Carers should

1. Encourage parents of a child with croup symptoms to take their child to their GP.

2. Alert other parents if their children have been exposed to a child suffering from croup. Maintain confidentiality.

Parents should

1. If the child is distressed, sit them upright and provide reassurance. Keeping the child calm helps relax the already narrow airways.

2. Encourage the child to drink plenty of fluids to help relax their vocal chords. If the child has a fever, the child may benefit from paracetamol which will help lower their temperature.

3. Some children get relief from being in a steamy room, such as a bathroom. This helps to relax the airways.

Child May Return to School or Child Care . . .

After 3 to 4 days most children will have recovered and the coughing will have subsided. If they feel well enough, they may return to school.

A Possible Cause of Coughing: Whooping Cough (Pertussis)

What You Should Know

Whooping cough (sometimes referred to as pertussis) is an infection of the lining of the airway. It is a highly contagious bacterial infection that spreads to others through droplets in the air from coughing and sneezing. The condition is known as whooping cough because the child will have a hacking cough, following by a sharp intake of breath that sounds like a "whoop".

Today in the United Kingdom, children are vaccinated against whooping cough at two, three, and four months, and again between age 3 and 5 before they start school. It is generally a mild illness in older children, but it can be life-threatening to infants because of breathing difficulties and the risk of pneumonia.

What You Should Look For

Whooping cough develops in stages, the early stage produces mild symptoms which are followed by a period of more severe symptoms before the child start to recover.

Early symptoms:

- Dry irritating cough
- Sneezing and runny nose
- Sore throat
- Slightly raised temperature
- Feeling generally unwell

Later symptoms:

- Bouts of coughing (12 to 15 per day)
- Coughing up thick phlegm
- Whoop sound caused by sharp breath following each cough
- Tiredness/red face from coughing

The early symptoms last for 1 to 2 weeks and the more severe symptoms of bouts of coughing usually only last a fortnight, but can continue for a couple of months.

What You Should Do

Carers and parents should

1. The child must see their general practitioner (GP) as soon as possible. The GP is obliged to inform the local health authorities.

2. Ensure that all children have received their immunisation programme according to current recommendations. Whooping cough is preventable by vaccination.

3. Monitor staff and children for respiratory signs or symptoms for 21 days after the last contact with an infected child.

Carers should

1. Encourage parents of a child with a prolonged cough to take the child to their GP.

2. Alert other parents if their children have been exposed to a child who is diagnosed with whooping cough. Encourage them to contact their GP. Maintain confidentiality.

3. Monitor staff for respiratory illness and recommend that they seek treatment if they develop a persistent cough.

Parents should

Have the child seen by their GP for prolonged cough.

Child May Return to School or Child Care . . .

The child may return to school 5 days after commencing a course of antibiotics. If the child was not prescribed antibiotics, they should wait until 3 weeks after intense coughing bouts end. Although coughing may continue long after the 3 weeks, it is unlikely the child will still be infectious.

Diarrhoea

What You Should Know

Diarrhoea is the passing of frequent, watery, less-formed stools. It is caused primarily by viruses. It also can be caused by bacterial or parasitic infections, some medications (especially antibiotics), changes in diet, and certain foods. It may resolve without treatment within a few days. If mild diarrhoea does not resolve within a few days or if there is blood in the diarrhoea, the child should be seen by a health care professional for a stool culture to determine if the diarrhoea is infectious.

What You Should Look For

- Frequent loose or watery stools compared to the child's normal pattern
- Nausea and vomiting
- Abdominal cramps
- Fever
- Headache
- Generally not feeling well
- Blood in the stool

What You Should Do

Carers and parents should

1. Not let children and adults who have diarrhoea handle food until after 48 hours of symptoms clearing up.

2. Call a health care professional if the child has any of the following:

   - Blood in stool
   - Frequent vomiting

- Abdominal pain
- Less frequent urination
- No tears when crying
- Loss of appetite for liquids
- High fever
- Frequent or persistent diarrhoea
- Dry, sticky mouth or tongue
- Weight loss
- Headache

Carers should

1. Notify parents.

2. Practise particularly careful and frequent hand washing, especially after using the toilet or handling soiled nappies, and before anything having to do with food preparation or eating.

3. Encourage the child to drink clear fluids regularly if you believe they are becoming dehydrated.

4. Offer food as soon as the child feels he/she can eat. Carbohydrate-rich foods, such as pasta, bread, or potatoes are particularly helpful.

Parents should

1. Take the child to their GP if the diarrhoea has not cleared up after 3 to 4 days.

Child May Return to School or Child Care . . .

- If cleared by a health professional after bloody diarrhoea and diarrhoea caused by certain bacteria (e.g., *Shigella, Salmonella, E. Coli* 0157:H7) or the parasite *Giardia lamblia.*
- When stool is contained in the toilet (for toilet-trained children).

- Even if stools stay loose, the child may return when the child seems well and the stool consistency has not changed for a week.
- When the child can participate in the program and the staff determine that they can care for the child without compromising their ability to care for the other children in the group.
- The child should be excluded from swimming practice for 2 weeks following the last episode of diarrhoea.

Possible Problem: Rotavirus Gastroenteritis

What You Should Know

Rotavirus is a virus that belongs to a family of viruses found worldwide. Rotavirus infections are extremely common in children. It is estimated that every child will have at least one rotavirus infection before they reach 5 years of age, with most infections occurring between 3 months and 3 years of age. Rotavirus is the leading cause of gastroenteritis in children.

The virus infects the stomach and intestines and is spread primarily by people not washing their hands adequately after using the toilet. The incubation period is 2 to 4 days and the child is contagious up to 3 weeks after the illness.

What You Should Look For

- Rapid onset diarrhoea
- Vomiting
- Abdominal pain
- Fever (38°C and over)
- Dehydration
- Generally lasts 3 to 8 days

What You Should Do

Carers and parents should

In most cases of gastroenteritis, the child's symptoms should resolve without treatment.

1. Routinely practice proper hand washing, especially after toileting or nappy changing, and before any contact with food or surfaces involved in preparing and serving food.

2. The most important factor during an episode of childhood gastroenteritis is to ensure that the child remains hydrated. You should encourage them to drink plenty of clear fluids, such as water or weak fruit squash.

3. Practice proper cleaning and disinfecting of surfaces. After surfaces are visibly clean, apply a disinfectant solution and leave it in contact with the surface for the time recommended on the product label.

4. Make an extra effort to practice frequent and correct hand washing, as well as cleaning and disinfecting of surfaces whenever an outbreak occurs.

5. The use of oral rehydration solutions are recommended and can be purchased from your local pharmacists without a prescription.

6. Notify all parents when an outbreak occurs so they can watch for symptoms and make an extra effort to prevent the spread of the illness in their families.

Carers should

Notify parents.

Parents should

1. As soon as your child's vomiting is under control, you should encourage them to start eating regularly. Food will not make the diarrhoea worse and the nutrients gained will be beneficial to help regain strength.

2. If your child has a fever or is in pain, paracetamol may help relieve these symptoms. Remember to always give the dosage according to the manufacturer's instructions.

3. The use of anti-diarrhoea medicine is not recommended for children under 12 years of age.

Child May Return to School or Child Care . . .

Children should not return to school or child care until 48 hours have passed since their last bout of diarrhoea and vomiting. A child should also refrain from swimming practice for 2 weeks following their last episode of diarrhoea.

Earache

Possible Problem: Otitis Externa

What You Should Know

Otitis externa causes inflammation and swelling of the external ear canal (the tube between the outer ear and the ear drum). It can be caused by an infection or by an allergic reaction to something that comes into contact with the external ear canal. In some cases, it is caused by water entering the ear canal. This is a condition known as swimmer's ear or surfer's ear.

The actual infection may be in one small place, for instance in the follicle of one hair root, or it may be widespread throughout the canal.

What You Should Look For

- Red, swollen outer ear
- Painful outer ear

- Itchiness or irritation
- Tenderness when opening the jaw
- Scaly skin in ear canal
- Discharge
- Some hearing loss

What You Should Do

Carers and parents should

1. Prevent the child from getting their affected ear wet, for example by wearing a shower cap while showering and bathing. Remove any discharge or debris by gently swabbing the ear with cotton wool, being careful not to damage it.

2. Encourage the child to remove anything from their affected ear that may be causing an allergic reaction, such as hearing aids, ear plugs, and earrings.

Carers should

1. Ensure parents are aware of condition and suggest they make an appointment with the child's GP.

Parents should

1. Remove any discharge or debris by gently swabbing the child's ear with cotton wool, being careful not to damage it and not pushing into the canal.

2. Encourage their child to not get soap or shampoo in their ears when showering or bathing.

3. Ensure that a child does not put things such as cotton buds, corners of towels, etc. into their ears.

4. Visit the child's GP to discuss any underlying skin condition that may aggravate the otitis externa, such as seborrhoeic dermatitis, psoriasis, or eczema. In some cases, antibiotics may be required.

5. If your child has a fever or is in pain, paracetamol may help relieve these symptoms. Remember to always give the dosage according to the manufacturer's instructions. If you are unsure, check with your GP, practice nurse, or pharmacists. Children under the age of 16 should not take aspirin.

Child May Return to School or Child Care . . .

- Exclusion for ear infection is not necessary unless the child is too ill to participate or requires too much care to allow carers to meet the needs of the other children.
- It would be advisable to curtail water-based activities unless bathing caps are worn.

Possible Problem: Otitis Media (Middle Ear Infection)

What You Should Know

An infection of the middle ear most often occurs when fluid or mucus accumulates in the middle ear space. The mucus can come from a cold, allergy, or some other irritant of the respiratory tract. Mucus collects more easily in small children because the Eustachian tube that normally drains the middle ear is small, more horizontal, and easily blocked. Most middle ear infections are caused by viruses and resolve themselves within 3 days without any intervention.

Acute otitis media is a short-term ear infection that often comes on suddenly, whereas chronic otitis media relates to ear infections which keep coming back or one infection that lasts for a very long time.

What You Should Look For

- Earache
- Fever

- Pain or irritability
- Difficulty hearing
- Blocked ears
- Drainage
- Swelling around ear

What You Should Do

Carers and parents should

1. Keep the child with an earache and fever well hydrated.

2. Prevent room air from becoming too dry. Dry air tends to dry out the secretions and make them thicker and harder to drain.

3. Ventilate indoor spaces with fresh outdoor air at least daily to reduce the concentration of germs in the air.

4. Follow the GP's instructions to take care of the ear infection.

5. Do not allow children to drink from a bottle while lying on their backs. This position allows fluids to enter the Eustachian tube, causing irritation that can make it easier for an ear infection to start.

6. Watch for hearing loss or speech problems in children with recurring ear infections.

Carers should

Notify parents.

Parents should

1. Follow carer's recommendations.

2. Call child's GP for advice if the child has earache.

3. If your child has a fever or is in pain, paracetamol may help relieve these symptoms. Remember to always give the dosage according to the manufacturer's instructions.

Child May Return to School or Child Care . . .

- Exclusion for ear infection is not necessary unless the child is too ill to participate or requires too much care to allow carers to meet the needs of the other children.
- A full return can occur when the child feels well enough to participate.

Eye Irritation/Pain

Possible Problem: Conjunctivitis

What You Should Know

Conjunctivitis is an inflammation (i.e., redness, swelling) of the thin tissue covering the white part of the eye and the inside of the eyelids. There are several kinds of conjunctivitis, including bacterial, viral, allergic, and chemical. The infectious form is easily spread when a person touches discharge from an infected eye on surfaces and then touches his or her own eye area.

What You Should Look For

- Red, irritated, or painful eye(s)
- Watering eyes
- Eyelids temporarily stuck together from encrusted discharge when child awakens from sleep
- Watery drainage is most likely viral conjunctivitis, a sign of allergy or chemical irritation
- Pus or yellow drainage is most likely bacterial conjunctivitis; may be treated with an antibiotic

What You Should Do

Carers and parents should

1. Clean drainage from child's eye(s) with clean tissue or gauze pad and warm water, as needed. Wipe each eye outward from inner corner.

2. Wash hands thoroughly and encourage child to do the same.

Carers should

1. Have children with irritated eyes get advice from a health professional about what to do.

2. Contact the health department about how to keep infectious conjunctivitis from spreading if more than one child has the infection.

3. Notify parents.

Parents should

1. Follow carer recommendations.

2. Contact the child's GP. Any condition that causes the eye to become red should be examined. However, it is unlikely that antibiotics will be prescribed as most conditions clear up themselves without intervention.

3. Apply antibiotic drops or ointment if prescribed.

Child May Return to School or Child Care . . .

The Health Protection Agency advises that it is not necessary to keep children home if they have a mild infectious illness, such as infective conjunctivitis. In some cases where an outbreak has occurred, the school or child care may advise to keep children at home.

Possible Problem: Stye

What You Should Know

A stye is an infection of an oil gland inside the eyelid that creates a swelling, usually near the eyelashes.

What You Should Look For

- Appears as a lump in the eyelid, which may or may not be painful.

What You Should Do

Carers and parents should

1. Apply a warm wash cloth to the eye as often and for as long as possible during the day.
2. Encourage child not to touch his or her eyes and particularly to not squeeze the painful lump.
3. Wash hands thoroughly and encourage child to do the same.

Carers should

Notify parents.

Parents should

1. Follow carer recommendations.
2. Call child's GP if no improvement.

Child May Return to School or Child Care . . .

No exclusion is necessary for a stye.

Fever

Possible Problem: Infection, Illness, Overheating, or Reaction to a Medication

What You Should Know

Fever alone is not harmful. When a child has an infection, raising the body temperature is part of the body's normal defences. However, rapid elevation of body temperature sometimes can set off a febrile seizure in young children. This type of seizure is usually outgrown by 6 years of age. Fever is not a reason to send a child home. It is a reason to check for a cause of the fever and to monitor the child's behaviour for other symptoms of illness. The normal temperature for a child is around 37°C. A child who has a temperature of 38°C or above is classed as having a fever.

What You Should Look For

- Flushed skin
- Tired
- Irritability
- Decreased activity
- Temperature of 38°C or above. The best way to record temperature in a child is by using an electronic thermometer in the armpit. Ear thermometer readings are sometimes helpful.

What You Should Do

Carers and parents should

1. Attempt to ascertain the cause of the fever. If it is due to overheating, the child should be moved to a cooler room and dressed in cool, loose clothing. Sponging the child (even with warm water) often causes them to become upset and then cry, which in turn raises their temperature.

2. If you suspect that the child has had a reaction to a medicine or immunization, first ensure they are dressed in cool, light clothing.

3. If you suspect the child to have an infection or illness, notify the parents and consider consulting a health care professional.

4. Get immediate medical advice for infants younger than 3 months of age with unexplained temperature elevations of 38°C. An infant aged 3 to 6 months with temperature elevations of 39°C must also receive immediate medical attention.

5. Wherever possible, encourage the child to drink plenty of clear fluids, such as water or weak fruit squash.

Carers should

Notify parents.

Parents should

1. Manage the problem that is causing the fever.

2. Give fever reducing medicines such as paracetamol. Some children are able to take ibuprofen as an alternative, however children under the age of 16 must not be given aspirin. Always give medications in accordance with the manufacturer's instructions and record the exact time of administration.

Child May Return to School or Child Care . . .

Fever is not a reason to exclude a child from child care.

Headache

What You Should Know

Most headaches are minor and are caused by overexertion or stress. A headache might signal the beginning of illness. It also might signal a vision problem.

What You Should Look For

- Tired and irritable
- Holding head

What You Should Do

Carers and parents should

1. Have the child rest in a quiet, darkened area.

2. Give any medication prescribed by the child's health care professional.

3. Notify health professional in case of sudden, severe headache with vomiting or a stiff neck that keeps the child from putting the chin down when asked to "look at your belly button". These symptoms might signal a life-threatening infection called meningitis.

Carers should

Report recurring headaches to parents.

Parents should

1. Have child rest in a quiet, darkened area.

2. Give medication if recommended by the child's health care professional.

3. Call child's health care professional for recurrent or severe headaches.

Child May Return to School or Child Care . . .

A headache is not a reason to exclude the child from care as long as the child can participate and does not require more care than the carers are able to provide.

Itching Scalp

Possible Problem: *Pediculus capitas* (Head Lice)

What You Should Know

Head lice is an infestation by a tiny parasitic insect on the scalp and hair and are common in children aged 7 to 8 years old. It is diagnosed by finding tiny yellow/white eggs, called nits, firmly attached to a shaft of hair; adult lice are harder to find. Nits can be found all along hair shafts and all over the head, but especially at the crown, the nape of the neck, and behind the ears.

Lice are transferred from person to person by crawling lice or through the sharing of personal items such as hats, combs, and brushes. It is not caused by uncleanliness. Lice cannot jump or fly and are not carried by cats or dogs.

All family members who have lice must be treated at the same time. Lice-killing shampoos are pesticides; therefore, use them according to the manufacturer's instructions. Combing out the hair with a special lice comb to remove nits and live lice is the most effective and safe approach, but it is very tedious. Household remedies do not work.

What You Should Look For

- Persistent itching on scalp
- Tiny red bites on scalp and on hairline
- Open sores and crusting

What You Should Do

Carers and parents should

1. Machine wash all washable items in hot water, followed by drying in the dryer, or send them to be dry cleaned. This includes bed linens, blankets, towels, clothing, jackets, and hats.

2. Use the high setting on the clothes dryer.

3. Place pillows and stuffed animals in dryer on hot setting for 30 minutes.

4. Place items that cannot be washed or dried in a closed plastic bag for 2 weeks.

5. Vacuum upholstered furniture, mattresses, rugs, car seats, and stuffed toys.

6. Do not use lice sprays.

Carers should

1. Notify the child's parents.

2. Notify all parents of a case of lice, but maintain confidentiality.

Parents should

1. Follow carer recommendations.

2. Treat with lice-killing shampoo as recommended by your pharmacist. Follow package directions and wear disposable gloves when applying shampoo.

3. Treat all family members who have lice at the same time.

4. Remove all nits and live lice with a small nit comb, available in most pharmacies, or with fingernails.

5. Check all family members' heads daily for 10 days.

6. Do not repeat treatment unless the product requires reapplication, and then do not do so again without consulting a health professional. Often, dandruff casts are mistaken for nits, or old empty nits (eggs) may be present but pose no problem.

7. Scrub hair brushes, combs, and hair accessories, and then soak them in very hot water for 10 minutes.

Child May Return to School or Child Care . . .

Although unpopular, head lice are not a reason to exclude a child from school or child care.

Measles

What You Should Know

Measles is a highly contagious and acute viral disease caused by the rubeola virus. Although there is a vaccine, outbreaks continue to occur among those who have not been protected by the vaccine. It is spread by direct contact with respiratory droplets (spread by sneezing or coughing). It is contagious from 1 to 2 days before the first signs or symptoms appear (usually 3 to 4 days before the rash) until 5 days after the appearance of the rash.

What You Should Look For

- Fever, cough, runny nose, and red, watery eyes
- Small greyish-white spots in mouth and throat
- Mild to severe temperature
- Irritability, aches, pains, and tiredness
- After 3 to 4 days, red-brown spots which usually start behind the ears before spreading to the neck, head, and after 2 to 3 days legs and body, often joining up and appearing bigger

What You Should Do

Carers and parents should

1. Observe child for other symptoms, such as eye or ear infections or diarrhoea. If any of these symptoms are present, contact a health care professional.

2. Practice proper hand washing.

3. Practice routine infection control measures.

Carers should

1. Notify parents and follow instructions from the health department.

2. Exclude any children who might be exposed to the infection and who have either weakened immune systems or have not received the MMR vaccine for any reason. These children must be excluded for 2 weeks after the last child in the outbreak breaks out in the measles rash.

Parents should

1. Notify their health care professional.

2. Keep their child's vaccines up-to-date. The first vaccination should be given at 13 months of age, with a booster given prior to starting school (usually 3 to 5 years old).

3. If your child has a fever or is in pain, paracetamol may help relieve these symptoms. Remember to always give the dosage according to the manufacturer's instructions. If you are unsure, check with your GP, practice nurse, or pharmacist. Children under the age of 16 should not take aspirin.

Child May Return to School or Child Care . . .

- At least five days after the beginning of the rash.
- When the child is able to participate and staff determine that they can care for the child without compromising their ability to care for the health and safety of the other children in the group.

Meningitis

What You Should Know

Meninigitis is an infection of the protective layers surrounding the brain and spinal cord. These layers, or meninges, once infected may become inflamed and swollen. The infection may be caused by either a virus or bacteria, with the latter causing the most serious, and sometimes lethal symptoms.

Viral meningitis is most common in babies under one year old, but can occur in any age range. The symptoms, often described as flu-like, are self-limiting and disappear in a few weeks.

Bacterial meningitis is a potentially fatal infection. It occurs most commonly in children under three years of age and in teenagers between 16 to 24 years of age. The number of cases of bacterial meningitis continues to drop as more and more parents ensure their children are properly vaccinated.

What You Should Look For

Viral Meningitis:

- Flu-like symptoms
- Headache
- Photophobia
- Fever
- Chills
- Muscle and joint ache
- Nausea and vomiting

Bacterial Meningitis:

- Fever
- Severe headache
- Drowsiness
- Confusion
- Photophobia
- Pain in hands, feet, arms, or legs
- Pale skin with blue lips
- Vomiting
- Fits or convulsions

- Stiff neck
- General irritability or inconsolability
- Blotchy rash that will not fade when pressed

What You Should Do

Carers and parents should

1. Call 9-9-9 or 1-1-2 immediately for a child who is drowsy, feverish, and displaying any of the symptoms.

2. The rash associated with meningitis (caused by the infection spreading into the blood stream) is a late sign and may not be present in all cases. The "glass test" is a simple way of assessing the seriousness of a rash. By pressing the glass against the skin it will be possible to see if the rash disappears under pressure. If it does not, immediate medical care should be sought.

Carers should

Inform the authorities if a child has been diagnosed with meningitis, as well as letting parents of other children know.

Parents should

1. Ensure their child is up-to-date with their immunization programme.

2. Have a low threshold for calling a health care professional for any feverish child who is irritable and appears generally unwell.

Child May Return to School or Child Care . . .

A child may return to school when fully recovered. There is no reason to exclude siblings and other close contacts of the child. However, it is necessary to contact the child's GP and the Health Protection Unit for advice on tracing contacts.

Mouth/Lip Sores

Possible Cause: Cold Sores (Herpes Simplex Virus)

What You Should Know

Herpes simplex virus is a viral disease that causes a variety of infections in different age groups. It is usually painful. Once someone is infected, the virus can become active again periodically. During the first infection, people carry the virus for at least a week and may continue to carry the virus for several weeks after signs or symptoms appear. People with recurrent infections carry the largest amount of virus for 3 to 4 days after signs or symptoms appear. The virus can be carried by people with no signs or symptoms of illness. This virus is spread by direct contact with the sore or by secretions from the sore that get on other surfaces, such as toys.

What You Should Look For

- Painful small fluid-filled blisters in mouth, on gums, or on lips
- Blisters that weep clear fluid and are slow to crust over
- Irritability
- Fever
- Tender, swollen lymph nodes

What You Should Do

Carers and parents should

1. Keep area of sores clean and dry.

2. Not touch an open cold sore.

3. Wash hands thoroughly whenever contact with infected material might have occurred, and also at routine times related to food handling, toileting, and contact with soiled surfaces.

4. Wash and disinfect mouthed toys and utensils that have come into contact with saliva or have been touched by children who are drooling and put fingers in their mouths.

Carers should

Notify parents, family members, and staff who may have been exposed so they can watch for symptoms.

Parents should

Follow carer recommendations.

Child May Return to School or Child Care . . .

- When an open sore has completely scabbed over or can be completely covered and when a child who has mouth sores and blisters is not drooling.
- The child is able to participate and staff determine that they can care for the child without compromising their ability to care for the health and safety of other children in the group.

Possible Cause: Hand, Foot, and Mouth Disease

What You Should Know

Hand, foot, and mouth disease is a common and usually mild viral infection that is extremely contagious. The illness is more common among young children than older children or adults. It is transmitted from person to person through respiratory secretions and faeces. The incubation period is 3 to 6 days. The illness commonly results in a fever and blisters in the child's mouth and on the palms and soles of the child's feet. The illness usually resolves on its own in about 1 week, but the virus can be present in faeces for several weeks after infection starts. The virus can be carried by people who seem well.

What You Should Look For

- Tiny blisters or ulcers in the mouth and blisters on the fingers, palms of hands, and the soles of feet.
- May see common cold signs or symptoms with fever, sore throat, runny nose, and cough.
- The most troublesome finding often are the blisters in the mouth, which make it difficult for the child to eat or drink.
- Other signs or symptoms, such as vomiting and diarrhoea, can occur.

What You Should Do

Carers and parents should

1. Report the infection to staff responsible for making decisions about care of ill children.

2. Encourage seeking of medical advice if the child seems very sick or uncomfortable.

3. Practice good hand-washing routines, especially after toileting or nappy changing.

Carers should

Encourage the child to drink plenty of fluids, to prevent dehydration. Water or weak fruit squash are ideal.

Parents should

1. Consult a medical professional if the child seems very ill or very uncomfortable.

2. Not break blisters on hands and feet; they heal better if not broken.

3. If your child has a fever or is in pain, paracetamol may help relieve these symptoms. Remember to always give the dosage according to the manufacturer's instructions. If you are unsure, check with your GP, practice nurse, or pharmacist. Children under the age of 16 should not take aspirin.

Child May Return to School or Child Care . . .

- No exclusion from child care is necessary unless the child is unable to participate and staff determine that they cannot care for the child without compromising their ability to care for the health and safety of the other children in the group.
- Note: Exclusion will not reduce disease transmission, because some children may carry the virus without becoming recognizably ill and the virus may be carried for weeks in the faeces after the child seems well.

Possible Cause: Thrush

What You Should Know

Thrush is a yeast infection in the mouth that seldom occurs in infants over 6 months of age. The fungus is widespread in the environment, especially in warm and moist tissues. The fungus causes disease when it overgrows healthy germs in the lining of the mouth. This infection is usually treated with antifungal medication.

What You Should Look For

White patches on the inside of cheeks and on gums and tongue.

What You Should Do

Carers and parents should

1. Wash hands thoroughly.

2. Carefully wash and disinfect all items that might reinfect child, such as teats, dummies, and teethers.

3. Do not allow babies to share teats, dummies, and teethers that have not been washed and disinfected.

4. Follow the instructions of the child's GP for medication and treatment to reduce the amount of yeast to levels that do not cause illness.

Carers should

Notify parents.

Parents should

Follow health care professional's and carer's recommendations.

Child May Return to School or Child Care . . .

Children with thrush do not need to be excluded from the group setting.

Nappy Rash

What You Should Know

Nappy rash commonly occurs when surfaces that are wet by urine or stool rub against the skin. Also, bacteria in the bowel react with urine to form ammonia, which may irritate and burn skin. Nappy rash can be painful.

What You Should Look For

- Redness
- Raw skin
- Red bumps
- Sores
- Cracking of skin in the nappy region

What You Should Do

Carers and parents should

1. Use commercially available disposable nappies with absorbent material that keeps the surface of the nappy that touches the child dry.

2. Change nappies often—checking hourly by the look, feel, or smell of the nappies through clothing, and by opening the nappy to look for wetness or faeces at least every 2 hours.

3. Wash nappy area with warm water only. Avoid using soaps as these will irritate the skin. Allow the area to dry completely.

4. Protect nappy area with over-the-counter ointments, such as zinc oxide or petroleum jelly, which act as moisture barriers.

5. Wash hands thoroughly after removing soiled nappies and clothing, even if gloves have been used during the changing.

6. Baby powder is not recommended.

Carers should

Notify parents.

Parents should

1. Leave your child's nappy off for as long as possible. This will allow them to stay dry and avoids contact with urine or faeces.

2. Contact the child's GP who may prescribe topical medicines to treat the rash.

Child May Return to School or Child Care . . .

The child need not be excluded from school or child care.

Rubella

What You Should Know

Rubella, also known as German Measles, is a highly contagious illness caused by a virus and is spread through droplets in the air from coughs and sneezes. The measles, mumps, and rubella (MMR) immunisation programme has had a huge impact on the number of cases in the United Kingdom (UK) and, despite some adverse publicity to the vaccination, the World Health Organisation and UK Department of Health still strongly recommend that all children should be vaccinated.

The incubation period is approximately 2 to 3 weeks and the child may have a rash for about a week.

What You Should Look For

- Red/pink rash of flat spots which usually starts behind the ears and spreads around the neck and head before spreading to the rest of the body in a couple of days. The spots start separated but may join-up as the rash spreads over the body.
- Swollen glands around the neck, jaw, and ears
- Fever
- Cold symptoms (runny nose, watery eyes, sore throat, and coughing)
- Irritability
- Apathy and poor appetite

What You Should Do

Carers and parents should

1. Whilst many of the symptoms are similar to other more serious rash illnesses, the condition usually presents as a more mild illness. If you are unsure, you should telephone a health care professional or the ambulance service immediately.

2. The child may lack energy and should be allowed to rest and recover accordingly. Offer plenty of fluids, particularly at the height of any fever.

3. No treatment is necessary for the rash, as it is caused by a virus. Antibiotics will not work and the rash should disappear by itself within about a week.

Carers should

Inform other parents of a potential outbreak and provide advice/information accordingly.

Parents should

1. If your child has a fever or is in pain, paracetamol may help relieve these symptoms. Remember to always give the dosage according to the manufacturer's instructions.

2. Ensure a child is adequately protected with the MMR vaccination and has the recommended boosters as they get older.

Child May Return to School or Child Care . . .

A child becomes infectious approximately 1 week before any rash appears which usually lasts for 5 days. A child should be kept away from school or child care for 5 days after the rash first appears. It is particularly important to avoid contact with pregnant women, as the virus may be potentially harmful to the unborn baby.

Sickle Cell Anaemia

What You Should Know

Sickle cell anaemia is an inherited (genetic) disease of the blood. Normally, oxygen is carried around the body by red blood cells; however, the usual round flexible red blood cells are replaced with sticky, rigid, crescent- or sickle-shaped cells. When sickle-shaped cells block small blood vessels, less blood can reach that part of the body, depriving vital oxygen to organs. This is termed a "sickling crisis".

The condition is most common in black British, Caribbean, and African communities, but as it is inherited it is possible for the gene to appear in any community.

What to Look For

A sickling crisis may be brought on by a number of conditions, such as dehydration, a cold, infection, or a lack of oxygen in your body. The severity of symptoms vary from person to person and include:

- Sudden onset of tiredness and apathy
- Headache
- Sudden difficulty with hearing or seeing
- Sudden paleness of skin or nail beds
- Severe abdominal pain
- Increasing pain in joints
- Fever
- Difficulty/painful breathing
- One-sided weakness
- Blood in urine
- In boys, a persistent and painful erection

What You Should Do

Carers and parents should

1. A lot of children with the condition are able to recognise the signs that a crisis is coming on. Be wary of this.

2. If a child who is known to have sickle cell anaemia demonstrates any of the signs or symptoms, call 9-9-9 or 1-1-2 immediately.

3. Minor crises may be helped with simple over-the-counter painkillers, but it is always best to seek medical care with a child.

4. Avoid exposure to very cold environments (out of season swimming, hill walking in inclement weather, etc.)

5. Encourage the child to drink plenty of fluid, especially water.

Carers should

Have a low threshold for calling the ambulance service.

Parents should

1. Consult a health care professional when any sign of infection is present. Early treatment may help stop a crisis from developing.

2. Encourage a healthy and active life for the child, but be wary about the conditions that may precipitate a crisis.

Child May Return to School or Child Care . . .

There is no reason for the child to be kept away from school or child care. A child who is generally unwell may be kept at home to rest and drink plenty of fluids and can return when feeling able to participate as normal.

Skin Eruptions and Rashes

Possible Cause: Chicken Pox

What You Should Know

Chicken pox is a highly contagious, common viral illness lasting approximately 1 week. The incubation period is about 14 to 16 days, occasionally as short as 10 days and as long as 21 days after contact. It is most contagious from 1 to 2 days before the rash appears until all the blisters have scabs and no new blisters are forming. Shared air or contact with body fluids from an infected person spreads the virus. Shingles is the recurrent form of the chicken pox virus in someone in whom the virus remains alive; it can cause illness from time to time throughout life.

What You Should Look For

- Rash of red bumps appears primarily on face and trunk as fluid-filled bubbles that break, weep, and scab.
- Rash can also appear on arms, legs, or any mucous membrane surface, such as inside the mouth, throat, eyes, and vagina.
- Fever
- Aching, painful muscles
- General malaise, headache
- Nausea, loss of appetite
- Itching

What You Should Do

Carers and parents should

1. Do not give aspirin products to children under 16 years of age.

2. Follow the advice of the child's health care professional for management of symptoms, such as use of paracetamol for fever and cool baths to control itching and prevent secondary infection from scratching.

3. Watch for chicken pox to develop in other family members or playmates for 3 weeks.

Carers should

1. Notify parents.

2. Notify health authorities when a case occurs in group care so outbreak measures can be started.

3. Be sure that anyone who has shingles (adult recurrence of the chicken pox virus) covers their blisters so that the virus shed from these sores does not spread to others.

Parents should

1. Encourage child to drink clear fluids.

2. Bathe child in cool water to relieve itching.

3. Some children may be more comfortable if their itchy spots are painted with a thin film of calamine lotion. Letting a child paint her own itchy spots may be particularly comforting.

4. Trim child's fingernails or put mittens on infants to prevent scratching, which can infect open lesions and lead to scarring.

5. Consult the child's health care professional if the child seems very uncomfortable or ill.

Child May Return to School or Child Care . . .

When all blisters have crusted, approximately 5 to 7 days.

Possible Cause: Heat Rash (Prickly Heat)

What You Should Know

Prickly heat is experienced mostly by infants and young children. It occurs during hot and humid weather, when production of a lot of sweat swells the tissues around the opening of the sweat glands, blocking the openings of the tubes that carry the sweat to the surface. This makes little red bumps around the sweat duct openings.

What You Should Look For

- Tiny red bumps in areas that tend to be moist
- Commonly seen in skin folds of neck and on upper chest, arms, legs, and nappy area

What You Should Do

Carers and parents should

1. Pay special attention to skin folds that stay wet with perspiration, urine, or drool.
2. Use cool water to remove body oil and sweat, and then dry the area.
3. Leave areas open to air, without clothing.
4. Use air conditioning or a fan blowing gently on child to keep the child cool.
5. Do not apply skin ointments.

Carers should

Notify parents.

Parents should

1. Follow carer recommendations.
2. Dress the child in clothing that keeps the skin cool and dry.

Child May Return to School or Child Care . . .

Child need not be excluded from school or child care.

Possible Cause: Impetigo

What You Should Know

Impetigo is a *streptococcal* or *staphylococcal* bacterial skin infection that can develop after an insect bite, cut, or other break in the skin. It can develop in any skin injury such as an insect bite, a cut, or irritation caused by a runny nose. Children can spread the infection to other parts of the body by scratching. They can also spread the germs to others in close contact by direct touching or touching a surface that another child touches. Impetigo can occur anytime, but is most common in warm weather when cuts and scrapes from outdoor play are likely to occur.

What You Should Look For

Red pimples or fluid-filled blisters or an oozing rash covered by crusted yellow scabs.

What You Should Do

Carers and parents should

1. Discourage scratching.

2. Trim fingernails.

3. Do not permit sharing of towels or face cloths.

4. Wash hands thoroughly.

5. Cover sores until they are healed.

6. Observe rash and note any improvement or worsening.

Carers should

1. Notify parents to watch for sores.

2. If the child cannot be picked up promptly, wash the affected area with soap and water and then cover any exposed sores until the parents can arrange to collect the child for treatment.

Parents should

1. Follow carer recommendations.

2. Call child's GP for a treatment plan, this usually involves an antibiotic cream.

3. Clean infected area with soap and water and try to gently remove crusty scabs.

4. Cover infected area loosely to allow airflow for healing and to prevent contact that would spread the infection to others or to other parts of the child's body.

Child May Return to School or Child Care . . .

- 48 hours after treatment is started with an antibiotic cream or oral antibiotic medication or when sores have crusted and healed.

- When the child is able to participate and staff determine that they can care for the child without compromising their ability to care for the health and safety of the other children in the group.

Possible Causes: Molluscum Contagiosum

What You Should Know

Molluscum contagiosum is a viral skin infection, very similar to warts. It is most common in pre-school children. It is fairly contagious and is easily spread through close contact and the sharing of towels, clothes, and even toys. It is not a serious condition.

What You Should Look For

- Small, soft wart-like lumps which may be white or flesh coloured. They often have a dimple on the top.
- Spots are usually no bigger than 5 mm in diameter. If squeezed, a white gunge can be expressed.
- Most commonly, the spots are found on the trunk, thighs, bottom, armpits, hands, or face and may become itchy.

What You Should Do

Carers and parents should

1. Molluscum contagiosum should not require treatment as it usually heals naturally. In some cases, the healing process can be sped up by squeezing out the gunge. This is best completed when the skin is soft, particularly after a bath.
2. Ensure that towels, linen, and other materials are washed frequently and not shared between an infected child and other children.
3. Promote hand washing amongst all children and adults.

Carers should

1. Notify parents if spots are noticed.

Parents should

1. Consult the child's GP if at all concerned about the nature of the spots or any delay in the healing process.

Child May Return to School or Child Care . . .

Children do not need to be excluded from school or child care.

Possible Cause: Mumps

What You Should Know

Mumps is a condition caused by a viral infection of the glands, which are located slightly below and in front of the ears.

It is passed from person to person by airborne droplets through coughing and sneezing. Mumps is a mild illness, but complications do occur in some situations. It usually takes between 2 and 3 weeks for the symptoms to develop with one or two glands swelling up. This often gives the child a hamster-like appearance. This may last around one week. A child may still be infectious for around 5 days after the swelling has disappeared.

What You Should Look For

- Swollen salivary glands, either on one or both sides
- Fever
- Sore throat
- Pain on swallowing or moving jaw
- Tiredness and apathy
- Abdominal pain

What You Should Do

Carers and parents should

1. Persuade all children to cough into a disposable tissue, or if a hand is used it should be washed immediately.

2. Encourage the child to drink plenty of cool fluids, such as water. However, drinks such a fruit juices should be avoided as they will stimulate the swollen salivary glands.

Carers should

1. Inform parents if the child becomes unwell at school and arrange collection.

2. Inform other parents if a child is known to have been recently diagnosed with mumps and has been attending school, particularly families with pregnant mothers.

Parents should

1. There is no cure for mumps. If your child has a fever or is in pain, paracetamol may help relieve these symptoms. Remember to always give the dosage according to the manufacturer's instructions.

Child May Return to School or Child Care . . .

Any child who appears to have mumps should refrain from going to school for at least five days from when the swelling was first noticed. After this time, the child should return when they feel healthy enough to take part in normal activities.

Possible Cause: Ringworm

What You Should Know

Ringworm is a fungal infection that can affect the body, feet, or scalp. It is mildly contagious. On the skin of the body or limbs, the infection causes round or oval, red, scaly patches with raised edges and a clear area in the centre. The fungus may grow between the toes causing cracking and peeling, this is often called athlete's foot. On the scalp, the fungus causes patchy areas of dandruff-like scaling with or without hair loss. Ringworm spreads from person to person by direct contact; by sharing combs, brushes, hats, hair ornaments, towels, clothing, or bedding; or by contact with infected people or surfaces contaminated by people who have a ringworm lesion. Skin infections are treated with an antifungal topical cream. Scalp infections require an oral medication that must be taken for weeks. It is no longer contagious once treatment is started.

What You Should Look For

- Red, circular patches with raised edges and a clear area in the centre
- Cracking and peeling of skin between toes
- Patchy areas of dandruff-like scaling with or without hair loss
- Redness and scaling of scalp with broken hairs or patches of hair loss

What You Should Do

Carers and parents should

1. Alert exposed staff and families to watch for symptoms.

2. Wash hands thoroughly and encourage child to do the same.

3. Make sure the child takes prescribed medication for the recommended time for the treatment to be effective.

4. Avoid sharing of dressing-up articles or other clothing unless the fabric is washed between users or disposed of after one person uses it.

Carers should

1. Notify parents to collect the child at the end of the program day and not return until treatment is started.

2. On arrival and by observation while children are in care, note any areas of skin or scalp that might be affected.

3. Restructure dressing-up play areas or any place where clothing or headgear is shared to ensure that the equipment is laundered between uses by different children.

Parents should

Follow the GP's recommended treatment plan.

Child May Return to School or Child Care . . .

Once treatment is started.

Possible Cause: Roseola

What You Should Know

Roseola is a viral illness occurring in young children between 6 and 24 months of age. The incubation period is 9 to 10 days. It is mildly contagious. One bout provides immunity.

What You Should Look For

- A persistent high fever (38 to 42°C or higher) for 3 to 7 days
- Fever may cause febrile convulsion
- Often the child is not very ill when the fever is present
- Red, raised rash lasting from hours to several days that becomes apparent the day the fever breaks—usually the fourth day

What You Should Do

Carers and parents should

1. Contact the child's GP or emergency services to discuss the symptoms. It is essential to rule out other causes of illness or rash which may be more serious.

2. Notify exposed family members and staff to watch for symptoms.

3. Inform and reassure parents about the nature of the illness and that once the rash appears, the child is on the way to being well.

Carers should

Notify parents.

Parents should

1. Help reduce the child's fever by giving paracetamol or ibuprofen (if your child can take it). Remember to always give the dosage according to the manufacturer's instructions.

2. Encourage the child to drink plenty of fluids and ensure they are dressed in light clothing and the room is kept at a comfortable, cool temperature.

Child May Return to School or Child Care . . .

The child does not need to be excluded if the child's fever is not accompanied by a behaviour change and if the child is able to participate and if staff determine that they can care for the child without compromising their ability to care for the health and safety of the other children in the group.

Possible Cause: Scabies

What You Should Know

Scabies is a parasitic infestation caused by mites that burrow under the superficial layer of skin. The incubation period is 4 to 6 weeks for people who have never had the condition before, and 1 to 4 days for those who have been infested previously. The faeces of the mites that are left under the skin cause intense itching. It may be diagnosed by the appearance of the rash or by a skin scraping in which the mite or egg is seen. The mites are transferred by person-to-person contact and by the sharing of bedding, towels, or clothing. The child and all family members must be treated at home at the same time with prescription mite-killing cream or lotion. Itching might last 2 to 4 weeks after treatment. Scabies affects people from all socioeconomic levels without regard to age or personal hygiene.

What You Should Look For

- Rash, severe itching (increased at night)
- Itchy red bumps or blisters found on skin folds between the fingers, toes, wrists, elbows, armpits, waistline, thighs, penis, abdomen, and lower buttocks
- Children younger than 2 years are likely to be infested on the head, neck, palms, and soles of feet or in a diffuse distribution over the body

What You Should Do

Carers and parents should

1. Machine wash all washable items in hot water (above 50°C), including bed linens, blankets, towels, clothing, jackets, and hats.

2. Use the high setting on the clothes dryer.

3. Place pillows and stuffed animals in a dryer on hot setting for 30 minutes.

4. Leave items that cannot be washed or dried in a closed plastic bag for at least 4 days.

5. Discourage child from scratching.

Carers should

1. Notify the family of the child with symptoms.

2. Notify exposed family members and staff to watch for symptoms.

Parents should

1. Follow carer recommendations.

2. For those infected for the first time, it is recommended to visit your GP who will be able to assess and hopefully rule out other more serious skin conditions. If someone else in the household has already been diagnosed with scabies, this may not be necessary.

3. Over the counter treatments are available for scabies and usually come in the form of topical creams. It is essential that every member of the household is treated, and all at the same time.

Child May Return to School or Child Care . . .

After treatment is completed (treatment usually requires application of a lotion that stays on the skin overnight and then is washed off).

Possible Cause: Scarlet Fever (Scarlatina)

What You Should Know

Scarlet fever is a streptococcal bacterial infection that causes a generalized illness with a rash. It is the same type of bacteria that causes strep throat, but is not more serious than strep throat. The incubation period is 2 to 4 days. It is contagious and spreads from person to person by direct contact or by inhaling tiny droplets of infected secretions from the nose. Many people carry the strep bacteria in their nose and throat and are not ill. When the strep bacteria takes over as the most common germ in the tissue and causes illness, it must be treated with an antibiotic.

What You Should Look For

- Rash does not normally spread to the face, however the cheeks often become flushed and leave a pale area around the mouth.

- Rash appears primarily on trunk and is most intense at underarms, on groin, behind the knees, and on the inner thighs.
- Rash is slightly raised fine bumps that make the skin feel like fine sandpaper.
- Painful sore throat in children over 3 years of age; persistent nasal discharge and foul odour from the mouth in children under 3 years of age.
- High fever
- Tongue has white coating that changes to the appearance of a strawberry after 4 to 5 days.
- Nausea, vomiting, and decreased appetite
- Swollen lymph nodes in the neck (swollen glands)
- Headache
- Skin peels after 1 week

What You Should Do

Carers and parents should

1. The child will need the condition diagnosed by a health care professional. Scarlet fever is a notifiable disease, thus it must be reported to the local health authority.

2. The child's GP will most likely prescribe a 10-day course of antibiotics. Ensure the child completes the whole course, even if they appear to recover before all of the medication has been taken.

3. Encourage child to drink clear fluids.

4. Wash hands thoroughly after caring for child to reduce chance of spreading infection to yourself and others.

Carers should

Notify parents of the child and the families who may have been exposed to the infection.

Parents should

1. Wash hands thoroughly after caring for child.

2. If your child has a fever or is in pain, paracetamol may help relieve these symptoms. Remember to always give the dosage according to the manufacturer's instructions.

Child May Return to School or Child Care . . .

Your child may return to school or child care once they have been taking antibiotics for at least 5 days. Make sure that if they do return, they are able to continue taking the medications whilst not at home.

Possible Cause: Slapped-Cheek Syndrome

What You Should Know

Slapped-cheek syndrome is a mild virus also known as Fifth Disease, as it is the fifth most common disease associated with a rash. Slapped-cheek syndrome is spread from person to person through the air through coughing, sneezing, and close contact. This indicates that it may spread rapidly through schools and nurseries. It is rarely transmitted through contact with blood containing the virus. The rash usually comes 1 to 3 weeks after the infection. The incubation period is 4 to 14 days, but may last up to 21 days. It is contagious until the appearance of the rash. It can be serious for an unborn child (a foetus) or for children with some chronic illnesses, such as sickle cell anaemia and thalassaemia, or with suppressed immune systems, such as leukaemia and AIDS patients. One bout of infection is believed to provide lifelong immunity. About half of all adults have already had the disease, and 90% have had it by the time they reach old age.

What You Should Look For

- Fever
- Muscle aches
- Joint pain

- Headache
- Red "slapped-cheek" rash
- Lacelike rash

What You Should Do

Carers and parents should

1. There is no vaccination for slapped-cheek syndrome. Approximately 20 to 30 per cent of cases have no symptoms at all.

2. Care for symptoms of illness according to the recommendations of the child's GP.

3. Notify all staff and parents because of possible health risks to unborn babies and to children with serious illnesses.

4. A pregnant woman who is exposed to slapped-cheek syndrome should consult her health care professional for the possibility of having a blood test to determine whether her baby is at risk.

Carers should

Notify parents and staff that slapped-cheek syndrome is common in childhood and that hand washing is the best protection from infection.

Parents should

1. Contact child's GP if the child has a chronic illness that makes the child especially vulnerable to infection.

If your child has a fever or is in pain, paracetamol may help relieve these symptoms. Remember to always give the dosage according to the manufacturer's instructions.

Child May Return to School or Child Care . . .

- Child need not be excluded from school or child care unless the child has sickle cell disease or a compromised immune system. Children with these conditions may shed large amounts of virus and become very ill.

- No exclusion is necessary if the child is able to participate and the staff determine that they can care for the child without compromising their ability to care for the health and safety of the other children in the group.

Sore Throat

Possible Cause: "Strep" Throat

What You Should Know

A strep throat is a *streptococcal* bacterial infection. It occurs much less often than a viral throat infection, but it requires treatment. The incubation period is 2 to 5 days. It is contagious and spreads from person to person by direct contact or by inhaling tiny droplets of infected secretions from the nose. Many people carry the strep bacteria in their nose and throat and are not ill. When the strep bacteria takes over as the most common germ in the tissue and causes illness, it must be treated with an antibiotic. A laboratory test is required to diagnose it with certainty.

What You Should Look For

Some of the following symptoms may be present:

- Sore throat
- Fever
- Stomachache
- Headache
- Swollen lymph nodes in neck
- Decreased appetite

Strep throat is much less likely if there is:

- Runny nose
- Cough
- Congestion

Children younger than 3 years rarely have a sore throat. Most commonly, these children have a persistent nasal discharge (which may be associated with a foul odour from the mouth), fever, irritability, and loss of appetite.

What You Should Do

Carers and parents should

1. Wash hands thoroughly after caring for child.

2. Do not allow child to share mouthed toys, dummies, bottles, cups, or eating utensils.

Carers should

Notify parents of the child and the families who may have been exposed to the infection.

Parents should

1. Contact the child's GP to obtain a diagnosis and treatment plan.

2. Complete entire course of antibiotic treatment to prevent relapse, even if child appears to recover quickly.

Child May Return to School or Child Care . . .

- 24 hours after antibiotic treatment has started and after any fever has subsided.
- When the child is able to participate and if staff determine that they can care for the child without compromising their ability to care for the health and safety of the other children in the group.

Possible Cause: Tonsillitis

What You Should Know

Tonsillitis is an infection of the tonsils (small glands at the back of the throat) which can be caused by either a virus or bacteria. Most cases are viral in origin and usually effect children between 5 and 15 years old.

The incubation period is usually 2 to 4 days and the infection is spread between children through both airborne droplets and hand contact, usually sneezing, coughing or saliva.

Classically, tonsillitis is characterized by a sore throat and a feeling of general malaise. However, in most cases the condition clears up without the need for antibiotics or other treatments.

What You Should Look For

- Sore throat
- Red, swollen tonsils
- White spots on tonsils
- Swollen glands in neck
- Fever
- Headache, apathy, tiredness

Sometimes younger children have swollen glands in their abdomen and may complain of stomachache.

What You Should Do

Carers and parents should

1. Wash hands thoroughly after caring for a child.

2. Do not allow child to share mouthed toys, dummies, bottles, cups, or eating utensils.

3. Encourage children to sneeze or cough into a paper tissue and dispose of it properly.

Carers should

Notify parents of the child and the families who have been exposed to the infection.

Parents should

1. Contact a health care professional to have the child's throat assessed. A swab may be taken to ascertain the exact cause. Although antibiotics are seldom required (most cases of tonsillitis resolve themselves), it is important to assess the tonsils for any complications, such as an abscess.

2. Help reduce the child's fever by giving paracetamol or ibuprofen (if your child can take it). Remember to always give the dosage according to the manufacturer's instructions.

3. Encourage the child to get plenty of rest and have plenty to eat and drink, even if it is painful to swallow.

Child May Return to School or Child Care . . .

There is no formal recommendation for the amount of time a child should be kept away from school or child care. It is advisable that whilst the child is unwell and is being encouraged to rest, that they should remain absent until symptoms have improved and they feel able to attend.

Possible Cause: Viral Sore Throat

What You Should Know

A viral sore throat is the most common cause of a sore throat. It is contagious, but it will get better without treatment. More than 90% of sore throats are viral.

What You Should Look For

A throat that feels raw.

What You Should Do

Carers and parents should

1. Encourage the child to drink fluids. Avoid very hot drinks or food, as this may irritate the child's throat. Cool, warm, or soft foods and drink may help alleviate some symptoms.

2. Wash hands thoroughly after caring for child.

3. Do not allow child to share mouthed toys, dummies, bottles, cups, or eating utensils.

Carers should

1. Notify parents about the child's illness.

2. If two or more children in the same group have the same symptoms, notify the families of the exposed children to watch for similar symptoms.

Parents should

1. Follow carer recommendations.

2. If your child has a fever or is in pain, paracetamol may help relieve these symptoms. Remember to always give the dosage according to the manufacturer's instructions.

3. Consult a health care professional about a sore throat that persists for more than 3 days.

Child May Return to School or Child Care . . .

Do not exclude unless the child cannot swallow, is drooling excessively, is having breathing difficulty, has fever with a behaviour change, or the child is unable to participate or if staff determine that they cannot care for the child without compromising their ability to care for the health and safety of the other children in the group.

Threadworms

What You Should Know

Threadworms (or pinworms) are caused by an intestinal parasitic worm. An infection is acquired by ingesting microscopic threadworm eggs. It is common among young children who often put their hands in their mouths and who are poor hand washers. Many children have threadworms without noticeable symptoms. It is highly contagious in a family or childcare setting, because it spreads to others when the child scratches the anal area, gets eggs under the fingernails, and then touches another child's food or other items that might be put in the mouth. It also spreads from eggs on pyjamas, linens, underpants, and so on. Threadworm eggs can survive on external surfaces for up to a fortnight.

Threadworms look like small pieces of while cotton (hence the name), but are quite difficult to see. The best time to observe the worms is at night or early morning when the females come out to lay eggs. A health care provider may take a swab from around the child's anus to confirm the diagnosis.

What You Should Look For

- Itching and irritation around the anal or vaginal area
- Itching is usually worse at night, which may stop the child from sleeping properly.
- In severe cases, the child may lose weight, have a decreased appetite, and be extremely irritable.

What You Should Do

Carers and parents should

1. Discourage scratching of the anal area.
2. Encourage the child to wash hands after using the toilet and before touching food or anything that goes into the mouth.

3. Encourage children to not bite their nails or suck their thumb.

4. Encourage girls to dry the vaginal area after urinating and both boys and girls to wipe faeces off the skin after bowel movements (wiping front to back).

5. Tight-fitting underwear worn at night may help prevent inadvertent scratching. Be careful to change the child into more comfortable underwear in the morning.

6. If threadworms are the problem, seek advice about treatment from the child's health care professional. Wash and disinfect toys and surfaces used for eating, toileting, hand washing, food preparation, and nappy changing whenever they are likely to have been soiled.

Carers should

1. Notify the child's parents.

2. If threadworms are suspected, suggest that staff and family members watch for symptoms and treat everyone accordingly.

Parents should

1. Consult the child's health care professional for testing and treatment.

2. Follow carer recommendations.

3. Trim the child's fingernails short.

4. Wash child's bed linen, clothing, and towels in hot water and dry on the high heat setting; do not shake items, because this will scatter the eggs.

Child May Return to School or Child Care . . .

Children do not need to be excluded from school or child care if they have threadworms. However, the school or care setting should be informed so that enhanced hygiene measures can be implemented.

Upper Respiratory Infection

Possible Cause: Common Cold

What You Should Know

An upper respiratory infection is a viral infection of the upper respiratory tract (nose, throat, ears, and eyes). The incubation period is between 2 to 14 days, and the child is contagious a few days before signs or symptoms appear and while clear runny secretions are present. It is spread by direct or close contact with mouth and nose secretions or through touching contaminated objects.

What You Should Look For

- Cough
- Sore or scratchy throat or tonsillitis
- Runny nose
- Sneezing or nasal discharge
- Watery eyes
- Mild fever (between 37 and 38.5°C)
- Earache that may come after the secretions from a cold thicken and block up the drainage tube that goes from inside the ear into the throat.

What You Should Do

Carers and parents should

- Practice good hand-washing techniques.
- Teach children to "give coughs and sneezes a cold shoulder" by using their shoulder or elbow to cover their noses and mouths when they cough or sneeze and do not have a facial tissue handy.

- Teach children to wash their hands after sneezing, coughing, or handling tissues.
- Dispose of facial tissues immediately.
- Disinfect surfaces that are touched frequently (toys, doorknobs, tables).
- Ventilate rooms with fresh outdoor air.

Carers should

Notify parents about practices to reduce the transmission of cold viruses.

Parents should

Follow carer's recommendations.

Child May Return to School or Child Care . . .

Child does not need to be excluded unless the child is unable to participate or if staff determine that they cannot care for the child without compromising their ability to care for the health and safety of the other children in the group.

Urination, Painful

Possible Cause: Urinary Tract Infection

What You Should Know

Most urinary tract infections are caused by bacteria. Urinary tract infections are more common in girls than boys because girls have a shorter tube that connects the bladder to the outside (the urethra). Also, in girls, this tube is close to the anus, and bacteria in stool can easily get into the opening to the urinary tract. Boys do not usually get urinary tract infections unless they have some other health problem. Among boys with a condition that predisposes them to urinary tract infection, those who are uncircumcised are more likely to develop a urinary tract infection.

What You Should Look For

- Pain when urinating
- Increased frequency of urinating
- Passing urine with an offensive odour or dark colour, sometimes containing blood
- Fever
- Loss of potty training
- Fussy or unsettled toilet behaviour
- Fever (38°C and above)
- Pain in abdomen

What You Should Do

Carers and parents should

1. Encourage children to drink enough fluids to keep their urine light yellow or clear like water. Very young children can learn that a dark urine colour means they need to drink more.

2. Teach girls to wipe only from front to back after toileting.

Carers should

Notify child's parents about any symptoms of urinary infection and ask that the family consult the child's health care professional.

Parents should

1. Follow carer recommendations.

2. Call child's health care professional promptly.

3. Have child give urine specimen for testing and be treated as appropriate to the condition that the health care professional diagnoses.

4. It is probable that the child will be prescribed a course of antibiotics. It is essential that the child completes the whole course, even if they appear well before all medication had been taken.

5. Avoid using bubble baths; these products are common causes of irritation of urinary and genital tissues that makes it easier for a urinary infection to start, especially in girls.

Child May Return to School or Child Care . . .

Child need not be excluded from school or child care if the child is able to participate and if staff determine that they can care for the child without compromising their ability to care for the health and safety of the other children in the group.

Immunisations

Many immunisations are given during a child's first year of life, and a general immunisation programme extends over their first five years. Continuing into adulthood, occasional 'boosters' are needed to help maintain the correct level of immunity to a wide range of diseases. Many of these diseases have devastating consequences and can leave a child severely disabled, or in some cases facing a fatal outcome. Cooperation with the programme and ensuring a child received the appropriate immunisations in a timely way is an excellent method of promoting good health to your child and avoiding potentially serious diseases. Participation in the programme also goes a long way in preventing further spread of diseases within communities both locally, nationally, and internationally.

The following table outlines the most common immunisations that are given to children in the United Kingdom, in line with the Department of Health's Green Book recommendations.

Age	Immunisations	Method of Immunisation
2 months	• Diptheria, Tetanus, Pertussis • Polio • Hib (Haemophilus influenza type b)	One injection
2 months	Pneumococcal Infection	One injection
3 months	• Diptheria, Tetanus, Pertussis • Polio • Hib (Haemophilus influenza type b)	One injection
3 months	Meningitis C	One injection
4 months	• Diptheria, Tetanus, Pertussis • Polio • Hib (Haemophilus influenza type b)	One injection
4 months	Meningitis C	One injection
4 months	Pneumococcal Infection	One injection
12 months	• Hib (Haemophilus influenza type b) • Meningitis C	One injection
13 months	Measles, Mumps, Rubella	One injection
13 months	Pneumococcal Infection	One injection
3 to 5 years	• Diphtheria, Tetanus, Pertussis • Polio	One injection
3 to 5 years	Measles, Mumps, Rubella	One injection
13 to 18 years	Diphtheria, Tetanus, Polio	One injection

Source: Data from Department of Health, "The UK Immunisation Programme," *The Green Book* (2006).

Infection Control in Schools and Child Care

The following table is a quick reference guide of conditions that may require a child to be kept home from school or child care, thus helping prevent the spread of infection to other children or staff. The guidelines are based on Health Protection Agency advice and are relevant to the United Kingdom. In other countries, the guidelines may differ slightly.

Condition	Recommended Period to be Kept Away From School or Child Care	Other Notes
Athletes Foot	None	• Athletes foot is not a serious condition. • Treatment is recommended.
Chicken Pox	5 days from onset of rash	See Vulnerable Children and Female Staff—Pregnancy
Conjunctivitis	None	If an outbreak occurs, consult Health Policy Unit
Diarrhoea and Vomiting	48 hours from last episode	Exclusion from swimming should be for 2 weeks following last episode of diarrhoea
Hand, Foot, and Mouth	None	None
Head Lice	None	Treatment is recommended only in cases where live lice have been seen.
Hepatitis A	None	None
Hepatitis B and C	None	None
Impetigo	Until lesions are crusted and healed	Antibiotic treatment by mouth may speed healing and reduce infectious period.
Measles*	5 days from onset of rash	Preventable by immunisation (MMR × 2 doses). See Female Staff—Pregnancy.
Meningitis*	Until recovered	There is no reason to exclude siblings or other close contacts.

Condition	Recommended Period to be Kept Away From School or Child Care	Other Notes
Molluscum Contagiosum	None	A self limiting condition.
Mumps*	Five days from onset of swollen glands	Preventable by immunisation (MMR × 2 doses).
Ringworm	Until treatment commenced	• Treatment is important and available from pharmacist. • Scalp treatment available from GP.
Roseola	None	None
Rubella*	5 days from onset of rash	Preventable by immunisation (MMR × 2 doses). See Female Staff—Pregnancy.
Scabies	Child can return after first treatment	• Two treatments 1 week apart. • Whole household should be treated.
Scarlet Fever*	5 days after commencing antibiotics	Antibiotic treatment recommended for affected child.
Slapped Cheek	None	See Vulnerable Children and Female Staff—Pregnancy.
Threadworms	None	Treatment is recommended for the child and household contacts.
Tonsillitis	None	There are many causes, but most are due to viruses and do not need antibiotics.
Warts and verrucas	None	Verrucae should be covered in swimming pools, gymnasiums, and changing rooms.
Whooping Cough*	5 days from commencing antibiotic treatment or 21 days from onset of illness if no antibiotic treatment.	• Preventable by vaccination. • After treatment non-infectious coughing may continue for many weeks.

*Notifiable disease. It is a statutory requirement that Doctors report a notifiable disease to the proper officer of the Local Authority. In addition organisations may be required, via locally agreed arrangements, to inform their local Health Protection Unit. Regulating bodies (eg, Office for Standards in Education [OfSted]) may wish to be informed.

Vulnerable Children

Some medical conditions make children more vulnerable to infections that would rarely be serious in a healthy child. Children who are more vulnerable to infections include those being treated for leukaemia or other cancers, those on high doses of steroids by mouth, and those with conditions which seriously reduce immunity. Schools and child cares will normally have been made aware of such children. These children are particularly vulnerable to chicken-pox and measles. If exposed to either of these illnesses, the parent/carer should be informed promptly and further medical advice should be sought. It may be advisable for these children to have additional immunisations (eg, pneumococcal and influenza).

Female Staff—Pregnancy

In general, if a pregnant woman develops a rash or is in direct contact with someone with a potentially infectious rash, it should be investigated by a doctor. The greatest risk to pregnant women from such infections comes from their own child/children rather than the workplace.

Chickenpox can affect the pregnancy if a woman has not already had the infection. If exposed early in pregnancy (first 20 weeks) or very late (last three weeks), the general practitioner (GP) and ante-natal carer should be informed promptly and a blood test should be done to check for immunity. Shingles is caused by the same virus as the chickenpox virus, therefore anyone who has not had chickenpox is potentially vulnerable to the infection if they have close contact with a case of shingles.

If a pregnant woman comes into contact with German Measles (Rubella) she should inform her GP and ante-natal carer immediately to ensure investigation. The infection may affect the developing baby if the woman is not immune and is exposed in early pregnancy. All female staff under the age of 25 years, working with young children should have evidence of two doses of MMR vaccine.

Adapted from Health Protection Agency, *Guidance on Infection Control in Schools and other Child Care Settings*.

First Aid Kit Contents

There is not a mandatory list of contents for a first aid kit. The suggested contents below are based on a combination of advice from the College of Paramedics, the Health and Safety Executive, the National Child Minding Association, the Pre-School Learning Alliance, and Guidance on First Aid for Schools document. Other dressings and products may be made available however this table suggests a minimum level of contents.

Item	Quantity
Disposable examination gloves	3 pairs
Sterile dressing, large (18cm × 18cm)	2
Sterile dressing, medium (12cm × 12cm)	6
Low adherent, absorbent dressing (10cm × 10cm)	6
Non woven swabs (10cm × 10cm)	6
Triangular bandage	4
Safety pins	6
Waterproof dressings (plasters)	20 assorted sizes
Eye pad dressing (60cm × 60cm)	2
Disposable scissors	1
Microporous adhesive tape (1.25cm × 5m)	1
Resuscitation face shield/valve device	1

Index

Italicized page locators indicate a figure; tables are noted with a *t*.

Photo Credits

Chapter 1
1-1 Robert Byron/Dreamstime.com

Chapter 2
Opener © SW Productions/Brand X Pictures/Getty Images; **2-4** © St. Bartholomew's Hospital, London/ Photo Researchers, Inc.; **2-6** © AbleStock; **2-7** © kristian sekulic/ShutterStock, Inc.

Chapter 3
Opener © David Young Wolff/PhotoEdit, Inc.; **3-3** Courtesy of Amanda Brandt

Chapter 4
Opener © Stockbyte; **4-1** Courtesy of Kimberly Smith/CDC; **4-2** © David E. Waid/ ShutterStock, Inc.; **4-4** © Katrina Brown/ ShutterStock, Inc.; **4-5** © Jonathan Noden-Wilkinson/ShutterStock, Inc.; **4-6** © E. M. Singletary, M.D. Used with permission; **4-9** © Sean Gladwell/ShutterStock, Inc.

Chapter 6
Opener © Medical-on-Line/Alamy Images

Chapter 8
Opener © Mandy Godbehear/ShutterStock, Inc.; **8-1** Courtesy of CDC; **8-2** Used with permission of Dey, L.P.

Chapter 9
Opener © Jonathan Plant/Alamy Images; **9-1** Reproduced with permission from *Emergency Care and Transportation of the Sick and Injured, Edition 7.* Rosemont, IL, American Academy of Orthopaedic Surgeons, 1999; **9-2A** Courtesy of Dr. Pratt/CDC; **9-2B** © Photos.com; **9-4A** © Joao Estevao A. Freitas (jefras)/ShutterStock, Inc.; **9-4B** © Petr Jilek/ Dreamstime.com; **page 139** Courtesy of James Gathany/CDC; **9-5** © Topix/Alamy Images; **9-6** © Anestis Rekkas/Alamy Images

Chapter 10
10-1 © Thomas Photography LLC/ Alamy Images; **10-2** © Joy Brown/Shutter-Stock, Inc.

Chapter 11
11-1 © Amy Walters/ShutterStock, Inc.

Chapter 12
Opener © Eugen Shevchenko/ ShutterStock, Inc.; **12-2** Courtesy of Neil Malcom Winkelmann

Chapter 13
Opener © Robert W. Ginn/PhotoEdit, Inc.

Chapter 15
Opener © Say Cheese Company/Brand X Pictures/Getty Images; **15-1** © Joseph/age fotostock

Unless otherwise indicated, all photographs are under copyright of Jones and Bartlett Publishers, LLC, courtesy of the Maryland Institute for Emergency Medical Services Systems.